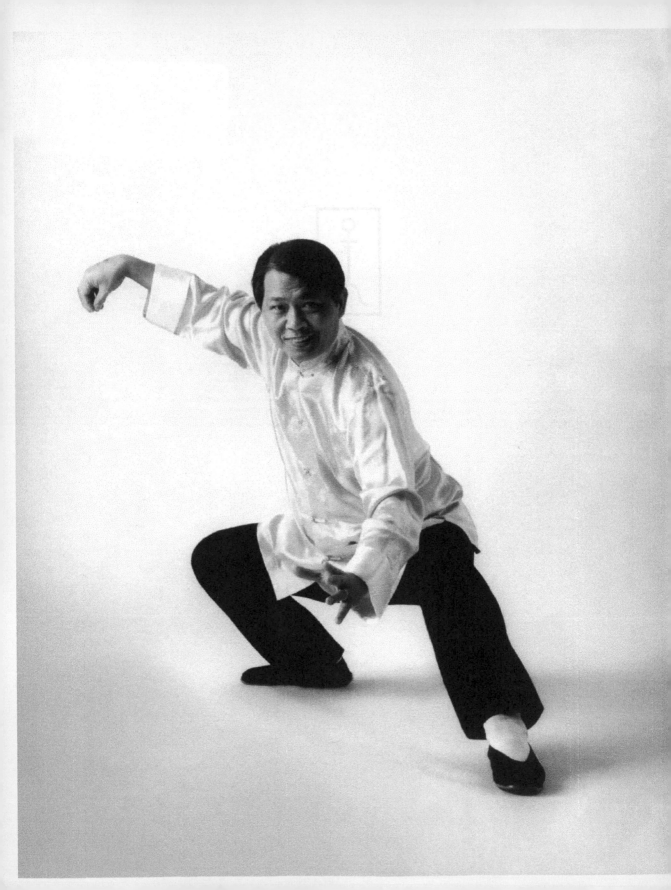

TAI CHI
FOR STAYING YOUNG

The Gentle Way to Health and Well-being

MASTER LAM Kam-Chuen

A FIRESIDE BOOK
PUBLISHED BY SIMON & SCHUSTER
NEW YORK LONDON TORONTO SYDNEY

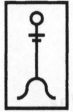

FIRESIDE
Rockefeller Center
1230 Avenue of the Americas
New York, NY 10020

FIRESIDE and colophon are registered trademarks
of Simon & Schuster, Inc.

For information regarding special discounts for bulk purchases,
please contact Simon & Schuster Special Sales at 1-800-456-6798
or business@simonandschuster.com

Designed by Bridget Morley

Manufactured in China
10 9 8 7 6 5 4 3 2 1

Library of Congress Cataloging-in-Publication data is available

ISBN: 978-0-7432-5504-2

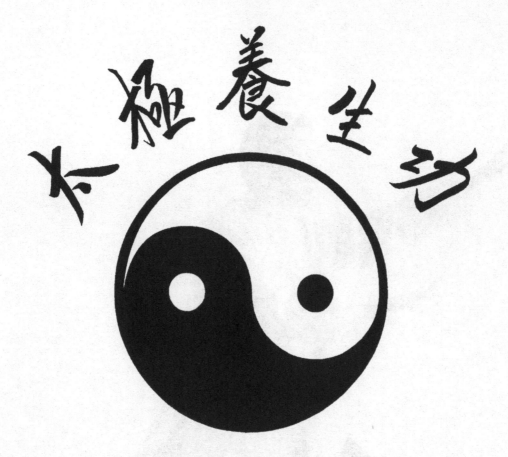

The Tai Chi symbol

The outer circle represents the totality of all existence. Within this circle, the interpenetrating forces of Yin and Yang are in balanced motion. Yin (black) and Yang (white) are the Way of heaven and earth, the mother and father of change and transformation. This potential is expressed in the small circle seed of Yang within the fullness of Yin and the seed of Yin within the fullness of Yang. All things and events grow and develop unceasingly.

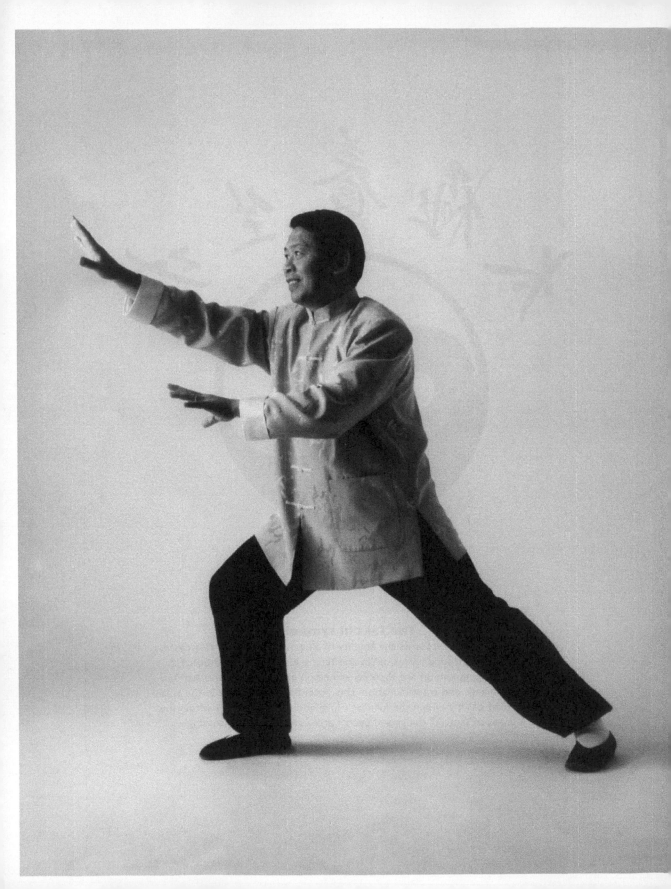

CONTENTS

Introduction

Every morning in the parks and gardens of China, people of all ages perform the ancient art of Tai Chi. This gentle way to health has been preserved over the centuries. Now it has spread worldwide, and is thought to be the most widely practised health exercise on the planet.

Regular Tai Chi practice strengthens your body, calms your mind and lifts your spirit. The combination of stillness and subtle movement, accompanied by natural breathing, relaxes and develops the whole person, improving physical and mental health.

One of the great attractions of Tai Chi is that it can be practised by people of all ages and at all stages of fitness. You do it at anytime and anywhere. You do not need special clothing, shoes or equipment. You can do it alone at home or with others. It is traditionally done standing but can also be adapted to a seated posture. Because all the exercise is done slowly and in a controlled way, there is less risk of injury. It is not competitive and everyone is encouraged to work at his or her own speed and level.

Tai Chi's healing power has been well known in Chinese culture for centuries. The carefully designed postures and flowing motions smooth the breathing and deepen the intake of oxygen into the lungs, thereby naturally releasing the tension we store in our bodies and encouraging improved circulation.

Hundreds of Tai Chi students, many of them senior citizens, gather in a London park to learn from Master Lam.

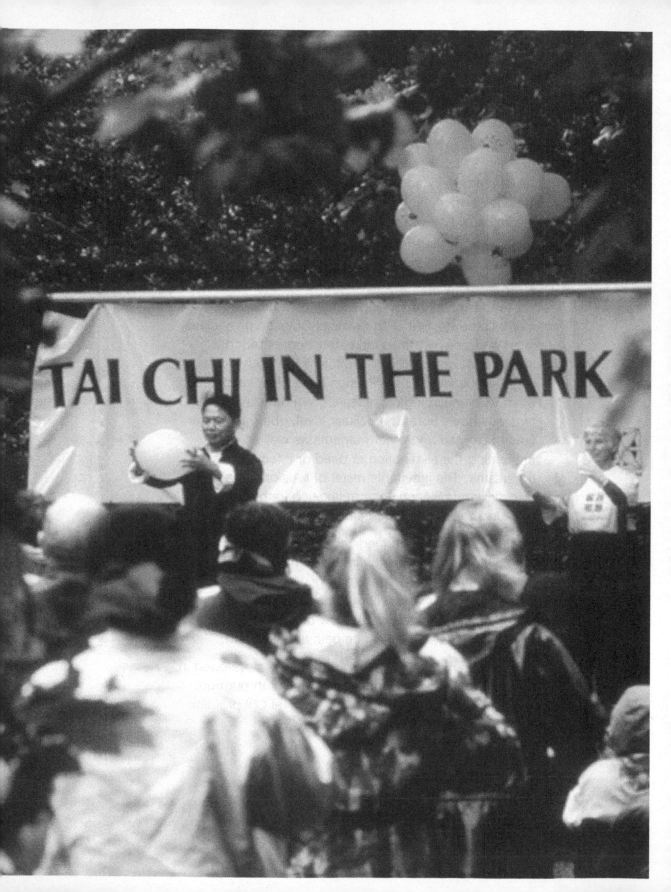

Complete energy training

Tai Chi (pronounced *tie chee)* is best translated as *moving harmony*. It is part of the remarkable system of health care developed over the many centuries of Chinese civilization. In classical Chinese medicine, one of the principal causes of bodily pain and dysfunction is tension.

We tend to think of tension merely as a problem of mental attitude. But to the earliest Chinese physicians mind and body were so intimately connected that mental tension could be locked into the body at it's most subtle level. Their findings have been validated by modern neurological research. We now know that tension shows up at the cellular level, obstructing the flow of oxygen and other nutrients as well as preventing the elimination of dead or infected organisms. The inevitable result of tension is pain, disorder and disease. Inner relaxation is therefore not a luxury. It is the key to health.

Health, in the Chinese medical tradition, depends on the flow of the vital energy in the human body. This energy is known in Chinese as *Chi*. When our Chi is flowing smoothly and without obstruction we experience health. When the flow of our Chi is blocked or diminished, we experience pain and ill health.

Tai Chi, like many other exercise systems developed in China, stimulates the smooth flow of Chi throughout your entire system. In this book, your Tai Chi practice is complemented by two other systems within the large family of Chi-enhancing exercises widely used in China. Exercises that promote the flow of Chi are called Chi Kung, literally meaning *internal energy exercise*. One of the most powerful of all Chi Kung systems is known as *Standing Like a Tree*. In Chinese, it is called *Zhan Zhuang* (pronounced *jam jong*). You are introduced to it in "The Golden Ball" section of this book, and each of the other sections of the book conclude with Zhan Zhuang Chi Kung positions.

The positions that you hold while Standing Like a Tree create just the right balance of muscular activity and relaxation needed to increase your internal energy levels. At the same time, the overall effect on your nervous system and your mind is to calm you down, thereby relieving stress.

You are also introduced in this book, in the section titled "The Eight Fine Treasures" to a set of exercises known in Chinese as *Ba Duan Jin*, also translated sometimes as *The Eight Pieces of Brocade*. These exercises are thought to have been developed by a famous Chinese general in the 12th century. They stretch and clear the internal energy paths (often called meridians). The movements are excellent for developing flexibility and strengthening muscle groups that are important for proper posture.

Understanding health

The circulation of energy is vital to health. If the flow of blood, lymph and other fluids within the body is restricted, the body begins to degenerate. Our tissue loses its softness. It dries out and becomes hard. The joints stiffen and the muscles ache. Our entire immune system is weakened as the flow of immune cells in the intercellular fluid slows and gets blocked.

Stress contributes to this degeneration. Many of the pressures of daily life mean that our whole system is on constant alert, even in sleep. We see the results around us every day: hypertension, migraines, asthma, all manner of aches and pains, some menstrual difficulties, depression and heart attacks. We tend to store the effects of stress in our musculature, as everyone with a stiff neck knows.

The gentle movements you will learn from this book slowly alternate contraction and release of all the major pairs of flexor and extensor muscles and many of the smaller, deeper muscles in the body that normally we rarely use. This work not only restores the natural flexibility of our musculature but also warms and massages our internal body tissue, thereby releasing and encouraging the flow of blood, lymph and intercellular fluid.

The inner relaxation helps our posture. The spinal muscles elongate. The ligaments become more supple and the spinal column eases. This is often noticeable in older people who take up these exercises after a period of relative inactivity.

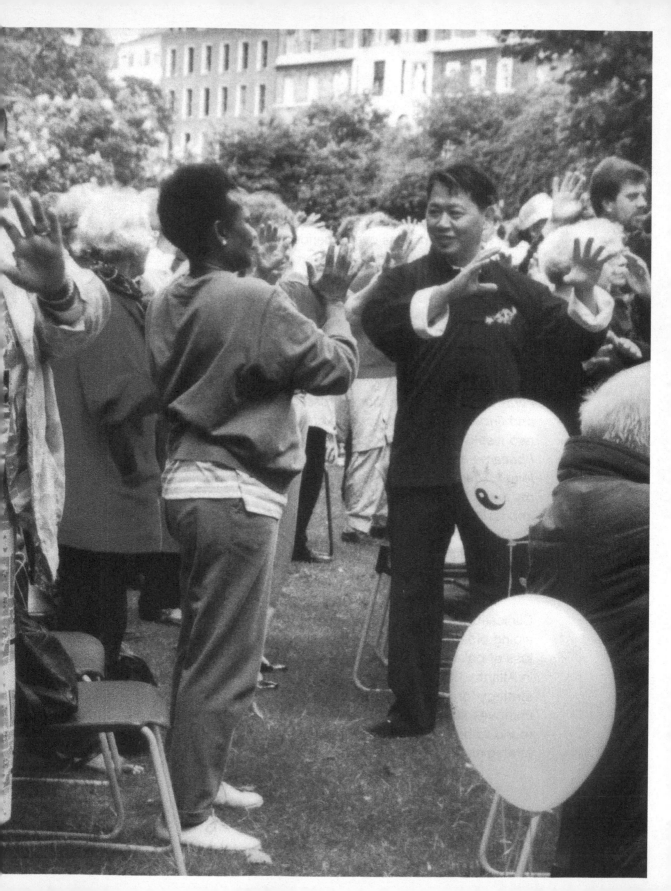

The Benefits

In a test of The Eight Fine Treasures (*Ba Duan Jin*) to which you are introduced in this book, a group of thirty office workers in the West was asked to keep a log of their experiences over a period of a month, during which they did the eight exercises daily. A sample entry reflects the experience of most of the participants in the test:

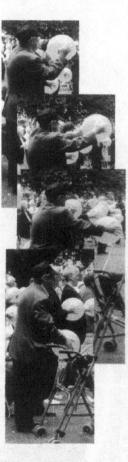

> " I had been working very long days with long stretches at the computer and had noticed that I was developing a lot of tension in my neck and shoulders. I was also tired, feeling quite stressed and irritable, and finding it harder to concentrate. During the first two weeks the physical discomforts lessened and I became aware of increasing suppleness in various joints. There seems to be a decrease in the pain in my lower back. Other forms of exercise have been impossible due to a risk of jarring the spine, but Ba Duan Jin seems to provide the right degree of gentle stretching, combined with deep breathing, to be beneficial."

Clinical tests point to the value of this exercise in aiding older practitioners with weakening of the bones, loss of balance and coordination. Research conducted in Atlanta, Georgia, showed that the most effective strategy for falls prevention was exercise that improves strength, mobility and flexibility. Tai Chi was found to be the most successful of all fall-prevention strategies tested.

THERAPEUTIC BENEFITS

Tai Chi and other Chinese health care systems are more frequently shown to be effective in the treatment of the following conditions:

Circulatory disorders
Anaemia
Heart failure
Strokes

Respiratory complaints
Asthma
Chronic bronchitis
Colds
Flu

Nervous disorders
Anxiety
Depression
Headaches
Insomnia
Migraines
Repetitive strain injury
Sadness
Stress

Endocrine problems
Diabetes

Reproductive disorders
Menstrual problems
Pre-menstrual tension

Digestive malfunctions
Constipation
Diarrhoea
Flatulence
Haemorrhoids
Heartburn
Indigestion
Irritable bowel syndrome

Immune deficiencies
Allergies
Glandular fever
HIV
ME

Musculo-skeletal difficulties
Backache
Breaks and fractures
Cramps
Muscular dystrophy
Osteoarthritis
Rheumatism
Rheumatoid arthritis
Sciatica
Soft tissue damage

The clinical results of tests conducted into Tai Chi and other systems that develop our internal energy are not surprising. Regular practice of these therapeutic exercises is excellent for raising your cardiorespiratory fitness if you are out of shape. Even more significant are results showing that when practitioners have been tested doing Tai Chi and cycling, their breathing efficiency and stroke volume (the amount of blood pumped with each heartbeat) are significantly higher while doing Tai Chi.

Research findings in both China and the West also point to the effect of this type of exercise on the human immune system. Studies have confirmed this particularly in older people. One of the most important cell groups in our bodies, the T-cell lymphocytes that act to kill virus-infected cells and cancerous cells, were shown to be 40 per cent higher in practitioners of Tai Chi than in a comparable control group. Other tests have shown increased production of immunoglobulin and a distinct drop in susceptibility to viral infections.

There is a relationship between the impact of this type of exercise on our physiology and its effect on our nervous system. Tests of the physiological impact show that people regularly manifest a reduced respiratory rate but with increased oxygen consumption, a lower rate of heartbeat but with increased stroke volume, and increased alertness but with negligible muscle tension. Other tests that measure the effect on the brain, show that these exercises have a deep calming effect, while heightening our alertness. Using an electroencephalogram to measure brain wave activity, doctors have reported that people initially registering brain waves of between 30 and 40 cycles per second (mid to high beta waves) have, after less than ten minutes of Tai Chi, registered the relaxed alpha wave pattern of as low as 10 cycles per second. Those who regularly practise this type of exercise can attest to their improved powers of concentration, coordination and inner balance.

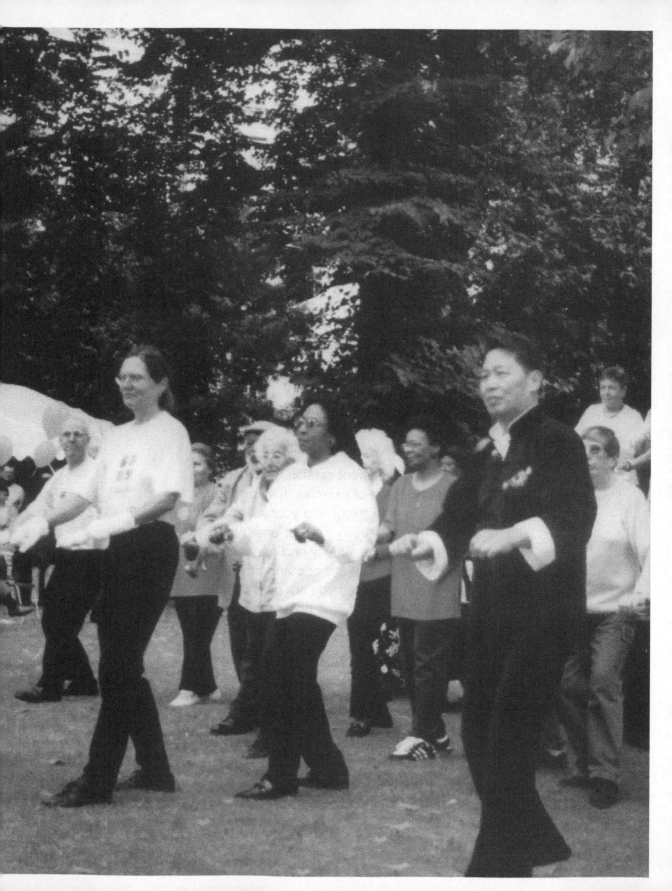

Relaxing and recuperating

Learning to relax is the essence of Tai Chi. The gentle movements and postures are designed to release tension. Please don't hurry or try to do more than you can. If any movement is difficult or painful, just do whatever you find comfortable. Rest calmly and then try the next exercise.

The movements are slow and smooth. When you stand, you are still but not stiff. Try to relax your lower back and slightly unlock your knees. When you extend your arms, don't straighten them completely. Your elbows should always be a little bent.

Everyone learns to do Tai Chi in their own way. Just follow the movements as accurately as you can and you will naturally develop your own ability.

Different people have different sensations when they start to practise this type of exercise. It's common to feel warm, even hot. You might find yourself shaking a little here and there, especially as your energy wakes up. After years of constant activity and nervous tension, it can be hard to sit still or stand still. But please try to remain still when you are practising Standing Like a Tree, even if your nose itches or you feel impatient.

If at any time you feel heat or pressure rushing to your head, start to have a headache, feel dizzy or faint, just circle both arms up to the level of your head and gently press them down in the air in front of you as if pressing a large ball down into a pool of water. This relieves pressure building up in your head. Repeat this calming movement six times. Each time, imagine you are standing in a swimming pool, up to your chest in water. You place your arms around the huge imaginary ball and slowly press it down into the water until you are holding it down below your navel. Then completely relax and rest, breathing naturally.

Sitting and lying

You can adapt many of the exercises in this book to do them sitting or lying. If it is not possible to reach above your head, you can try doing the same exercise out in front or to the side. You can try moving one arm or hand at a time, if it is not possible to do both at the same time.

You can practise The Golden Ball (pages 46–67) while lying down. These exercises can be extremely helpful if you are recovering from an illness or an operation. The two best exercises for restoring your energy are Holding the belly (pages 64–65) and Gathering your energy (pages 44–45). These can be done in bed for a few minutes at various times throughout the day.

Practising in nature

You can practise Tai Chi outdoors in a garden, on a balcony or in a local park. This is the way Tai Chi has been practised in China for centuries. You will feel refreshed by the air around you. But don't practise outdoors when it is windy or raining. If you find it difficult to go outdoors for any reason, try to have a source of fresh air in the room where you do your exercises. If it is not possible to open a window, at least try to practise in a room where the air is not too stale.

If you go outside to do your exercises, there are some tips that will help you get the maximum benefit. Try to stand with the sun shining on your back. This enables the sun's energy to radiate directly on the area around your kidneys and has the effect of energizing your body's entire Chi system. In any case, don't stand with the sun shining in your eyes. This will increase your nervous tension as your eye muscles and optic nerves work to protect you from the glare.

Practising in a garden or park where there are trees is wonderful. Trees are among the great powerhouses of nature and the energy they radiate is extremely powerful. The presence of trees is a tremendous support for your practice, stabilizing and calming you with their protective power.

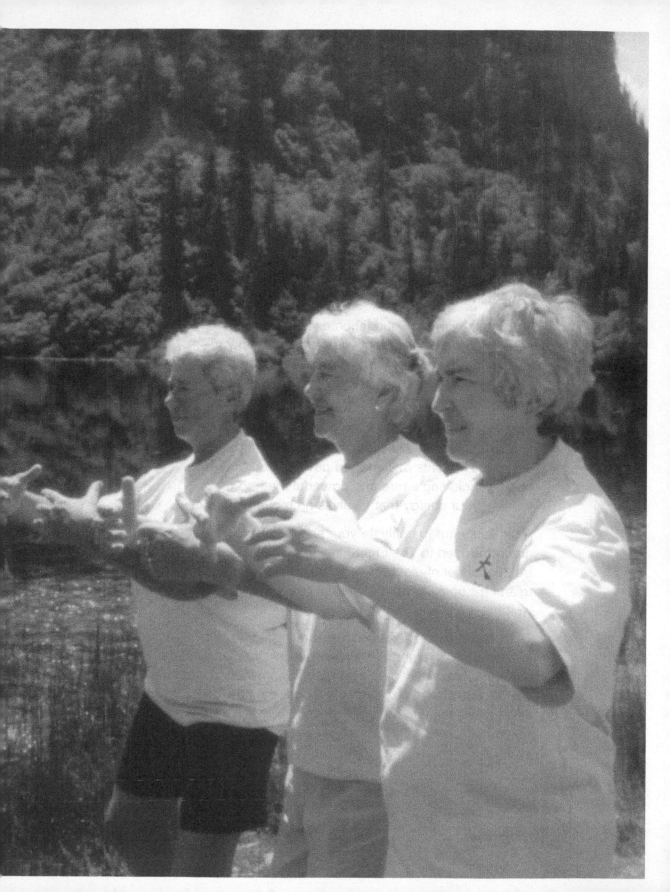

How to use this book

This book introduces you to three methods of energy cultivation, providing you with an integrated system of exercise and health care that will enrich your life. What you will learn is suitable for people at any stage in their lives, but this book is particularly designed to provide a style of exercise that is completely safe for people in their later years.

You begin with the Foundation exercises. These consist of a short series of warm ups, to help you relax and stretch before you start. It is important always to practise the Foundation exercises each day, before doing any of the other exercises in this book.

The Foundation exercises are followed by The Golden Ball exercises. This section introduces you to a short set of movements designed to develop your internal energy, including a rare and powerful method of training your energy that involves no movement at all.

After you learn to cultivate your energy in this way, you are introduced to The Eight Fine Treasures. This is a traditional set of eight movements that are particularly useful for opening up the internal pathways through which energy flows in the body.

Then comes a section titled Moving Harmony. This instructs you in eight of the classical Tai Chi movements which, when practised in conjunction with the previous training, will greatly boost the flow of energy throughout your entire body.

Finally, the book ends with a short section, Cooling Down. The set of cooling down exercises in this section should be practised by everyone, regardless of your age or fitness, to conclude your Tai Chi training.

Try doing your Tai Chi in the morning. It helps to get the day off to a good start. You can wear anything comfortable with flat shoes or socks.

If you do Tai Chi before breakfast, then drink a little warm water (not tea or coffee) before you start. You can have your breakfast any time afterward. If you have breakfast first, then allow a short gap before you start your training.

What should you do each day? Here's a simple tip for beginners. First do The Foundations. That will take between five and ten minutes. Then go straight on to practise The Golden Ball – the eight movements and standing posture shown on pages 46–67. That will take you roughly fifteen minutes. Then finish off with the Cooling Down routine on pages 112–119. That will take a minute or two. So your daily practice will last no longer than half an hour, and will be among the best time spent during your day.

Once you are familiar with the exercises and postures throughout this book, you can develop a daily routine that works best for you. There are suggested daily exercise routines on pages 120–123.

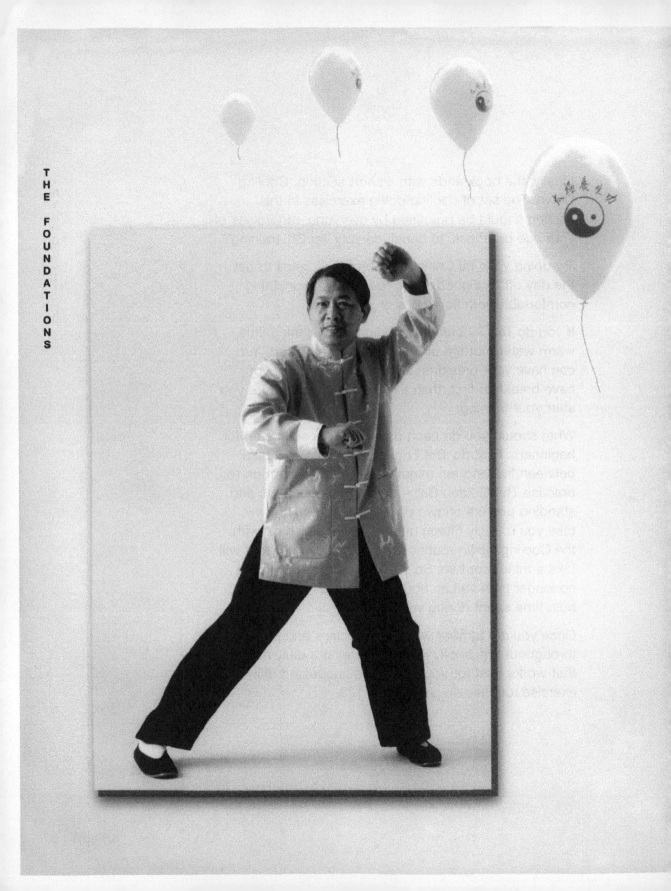

THE FOUNDATIONS

1   Warming up

Your daily Tai Chi begins with warming up. Take your time with these simple opening practices, to relax your body and stimulate the gentle flow of your energy.

This first exercise brings your energy out to the palms and fingertips of both hands. Most people experience the effect immediately.

Simply place your hands together and rub them together vigorously for about a minute. Try to feel that your fingers and fingertips are rubbing against each other as well as your palms.

Then use your hands to massage any area of your body where you have an ache or pain, or any joints that are stiff. Just move your hands firmly around the area with gentle pressure.

You can also give yourself a little "Chi facial" this way. Gently rub your hands over your eyes, ears and face as if washing yourself. Try feeling the effect of holding your palms over your closed eyes for a few seconds, then over your ears and finally over the back of your neck.

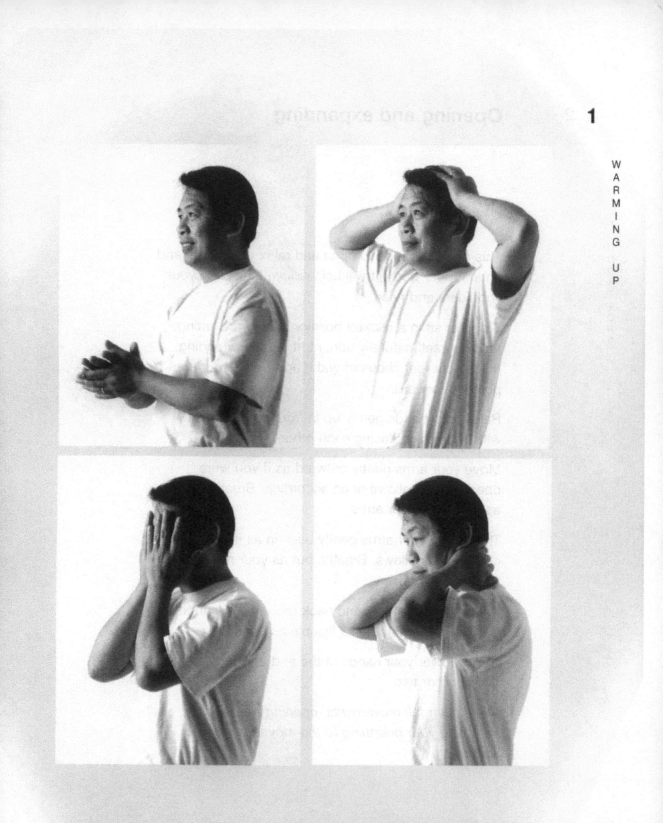

Opening and expanding

This exercise helps to open and relax your chest and entire upper body. It will help relieve tension in your shoulders and neck.

Stand or sit in a relaxed position. If you are sitting, hold yourself naturally upright. If you are standing, place your feet shoulder width apart with your toes pointing forward.

Raise your hands gently up in front of your chest with your palms facing each other.

Move your arms gently outward as if you were opening the bellows of an accordion. Breathe in as you open your arms.

Then bring your arms gently back in as if you were closing the bellows. Breathe out as your arms come toward each other.

Keep your shoulders and neck relaxed throughout and let your wrists be as flexible as possible.

Gently lower your hands at the end and pause for a second or two.

Make eight full movements, opening and closing, matching your breathing to the movement of the accordion.

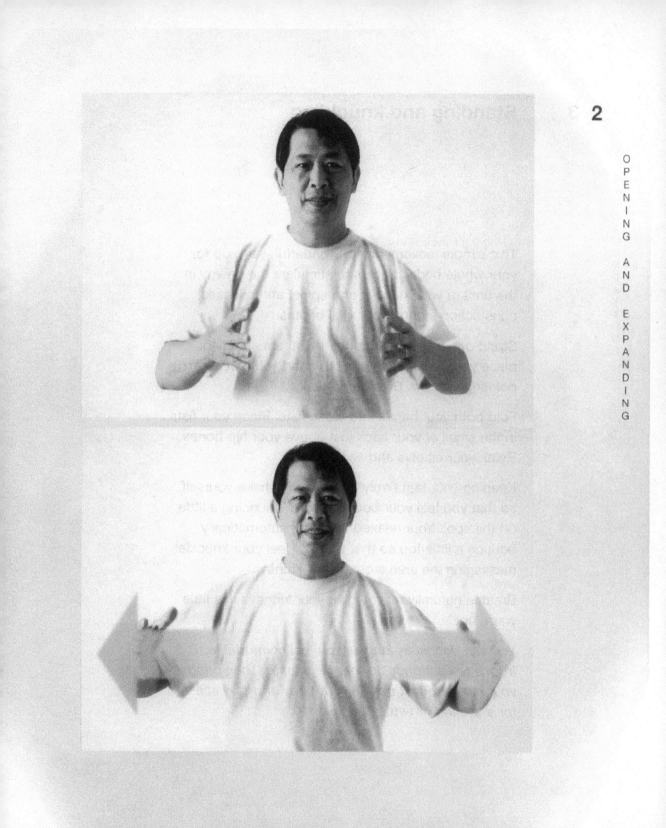

Standing and knuckling

This simple movement is a wonderful warm up for your whole body. It helps to stimulate the energy in the area of your kidneys and spine, and releases constriction around your vital organs.

Stand or sit naturally upright. If you are standing, place your feet shoulder width apart with your feet pointing forward. Breathe naturally.

Fold both your hands into loose fists. Place your fists in the small of your back just above your hip bones. Relax your elbows and shoulders.

Keeping your feet firmly on the floor, shake yourself so that you feel your body naturally bouncing a little on the spot. Your relaxed arms will automatically bounce a little too so that you can feel your knuckles massaging the area around your kidneys.

Breathe naturally as you give your kidneys this little warm up.

You can do this as long as you feel comfortable, from a few seconds up to a full minute. Then bring your hands to rest beside your body and stay still for a second or two.

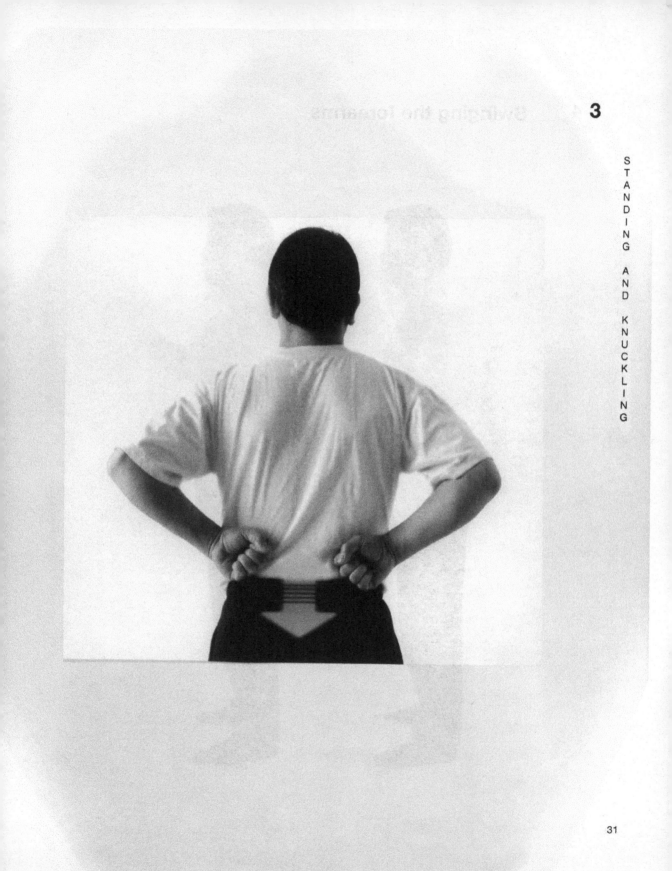

Swinging the forearms

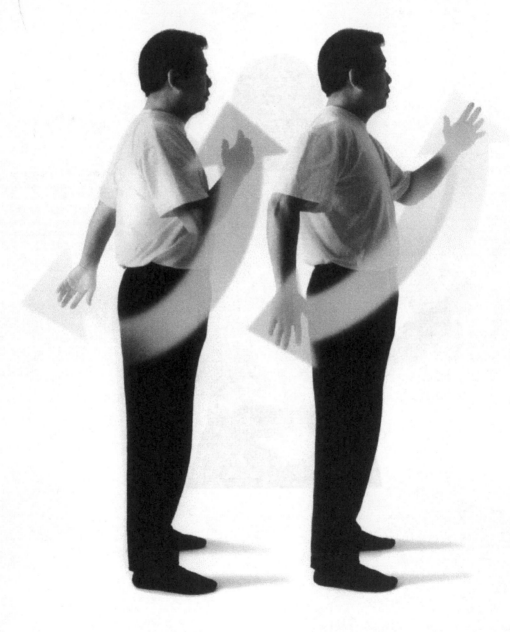

This exercise and the rest of the movements and positions in this part of the book are the foundation practices you should do every day, after completing the daily routine on pages 26–31. The foundation practices start to open up the energy pathways in your body and build up your energy levels.

This first foundation practice helps to release stiffness in your neck and shoulders and relax the musculature of your entire upper body.

It is probably easiest to do this exercise standing. Place your feet shoulder width apart with your toes pointing straight forward.

Relax your neck, shoulders and chest.

Look forward.

Swing your forearms briskly up and down by your sides. Your hands can come up as high as your shoulders and swing back beside you as far as they naturally can.

Keep your hands relaxed and open, but not limp.

Breathe naturally.

Try doing at least 30 swings.

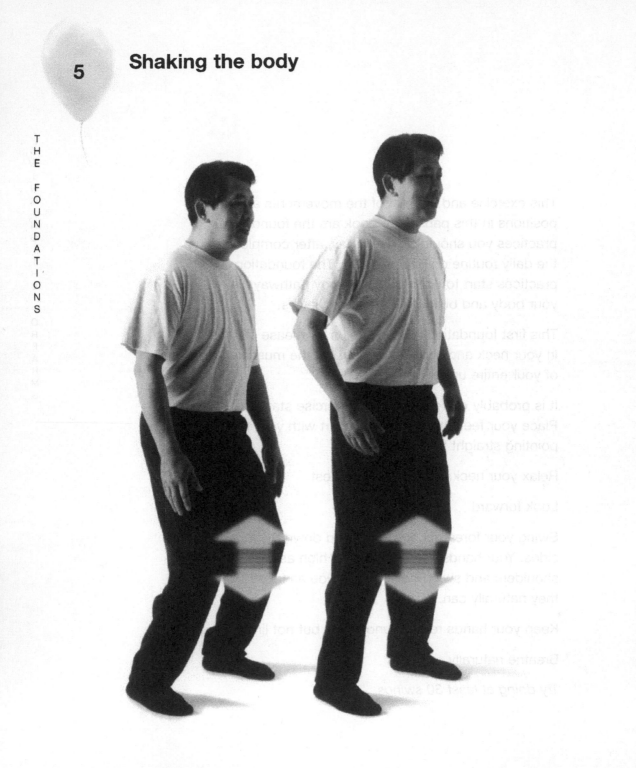

5 Shaking the body

This simple exercise has a wonderful effect on your circulation, is powerfully relaxing and strengthens your legs. The relaxed shake lets your major internal organs bounce a little inside you, giving them a wonderful internal massage. It is a great way of relieving tension and improving the flow of your innermost energy.

Stand with your feet shoulder width apart and your toes pointing straight forward.

Let your arms and hands hang loosely down by your sides.

Relax your elbows and shoulders.

Breathe in.

Use your knees to bounce your body up and down, as if you were riding a horse. You could also imagine that you are bouncing up and down on a trampoline, with your body loose and very relaxed – but of course your feet remain firmly on the ground.

Breathe naturally as you shake.

Try continuing this movement for up to a full minute.

6   Swimming on land

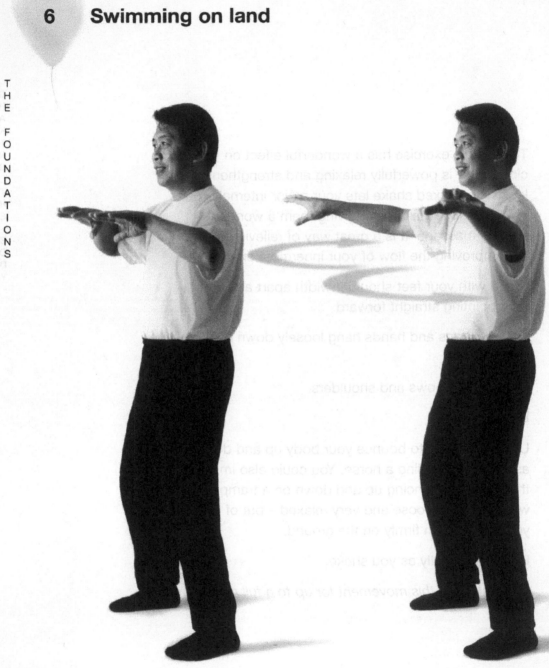

Stand or sit naturally. If you are standing, have your feet shoulder width apart with your toes pointing straight forward. Try sinking down a little, as if you were starting to sit down. Allow your knees to bend slightly as you do this, but be careful not to let them go forward over your toes.

Raise your hands gently up to chest height as if you were about to begin to swim using the breaststroke. Breathe in.

Extend your arms forward as if you were moving ahead in the water. Keep your movement smooth and calm. As your arms move forward, breathe out. Keep looking forward with your head up.

As in the breaststroke, your arms move apart from each other after they extend forward and then circle back in toward your chest. Breathe in as your arms come back to your chest.

Try to make eight complete strokes. Gently lower your arms and stay still for a second or two.

7 Standing in Wu Chi

This is the foundation position of all the Chi Kung
practices to which you are introduced in this book.
It is known in Chinese as Wu Chi (pronounced *woo
chee*). It is usually translated as the *position of
primal energy.*

Stand still with your feel shoulder width apart and
your feet pointing straight forward. Relax your knees.

Let your belly and hips relax.

Slightly sink your chest inward. Let your shoulders
naturally ease downward.

Let your arms hang loosely by your sides. Your fingers
should be slightly apart, naturally curved.

Lower your chin a little and relax your neck.

Look forward and slightly downward. Your eyes
are open.

Breathe calmly through your nose.

A gentle smile will help release subtle tensions
inside you.

7

Try to align yourself so that there is a straight line from the top of your head to the midpoint between your feet. You can use a mirror to check your posture at first.

Check that your head is not tilted to one side or the other.

Make sure your weight is spread evenly between your right and left leg. Begin with standing still for a minute or two. You might feel itchy, impatient or irritated, this is simply your nervous system reacting to your stillness. Remain calmly in place without moving, like a tree.

Standing and opening

This posture is the next stage in your Chi Kung training. There is a subtle difference between this position and Standing in Wu Chi (see page 38). If you follow the instructions carefully you will start to notice the different effect it has on your internal energy.

Begin by Standing in Wu Chi.

Your feet are shoulder width apart, with your knees gently unlocked, and your feet facing straight forward.

Your arms are loosely by your sides, with your hands gently opened.

Keeping your shoulders and chest completely relaxed, slowly open your elbows out to the sides. The movement is gentle and not extreme. You feel as if you are softly curving your arms away from your body.

Your hands remain by your side.

Breathe naturally through your nose.

Try remaining in this position, without moving, for a minute or two. Try not to move, allowing your internal energy to find its way throughout your body as it rests in stillness.

*Inner relaxation is the secret
of all health and well-being.
As you practise the postures and
movements in this book, your
inner work is to relax whether you
are standing still or moving.*

*You can then carry this inner
relaxation with you throughout
the day, whatever you are doing.*

9　Relaxing

Standing still in these positions calms your nervous system. This inner relaxation is vital to your health and well-being. If your nervous system is agitated, the flow of energy throughout your body will be seriously impeded.

As you stand in the two positions you have been shown on pages 38–41, follow this inner relaxation sequence while remaining still.

Bring your attention to the area of your eyes. Release any tension you may be holding in the skin or muscles. If your eyes feel tired, imagine you are releasing the pressure in your eyeballs.

Bring your attention to your jaw and make sure you are not clenching your teeth. Relax your tongue.

Let this sense of relaxation flow down your neck and over your shoulders. Allow each shoulder to sink down, releasing any tightness. Your arms will tend naturally to slide slightly down as you relax.

Release tension in your chest by breathing gently out.

9

Imagine you are standing under a warm shower. As the water cascades down your back, feel it washing away any tension in your back, as if dried mud were being softened and washed away by the water.

Feel the weight of your body sinking down through the soles of your feet.

Finally, imagine a fine golden cord supporting you from the top of your head. It stretches up into the heavens, gently suspending you. Remain still, repeating this inner relaxation as you stand.

10 Gathering your energy

This position seals your energy into the inner reservoir in your lower abdomen. It is always used at the end of any Chi Kung session as the concluding posture.

Place your right palm calmly on your belly, with your palm resting against your abdomen just below your navel.

Place your left palm comfortably on top of the back of your right hand.

Stand still, feeling the warmth of your hands and the energy in your belly.

Breathe naturally.

As you stand, your feet rest securely on the earth. Your upper body is relaxed, without tension. Your hands are calmly collected over your belly.

Remain in this relaxed position for a minute or two.

10

You can use this rejuvenating exercise at any time during your day. It calms your nervous system and refreshes your energy. You will find it helpful if you are feeling stressed or fatigued during the day. At night, if you have trouble sleeping, you can experiment with this position lying in bed. It will gather your scattered energy and help you settle down for sleep.

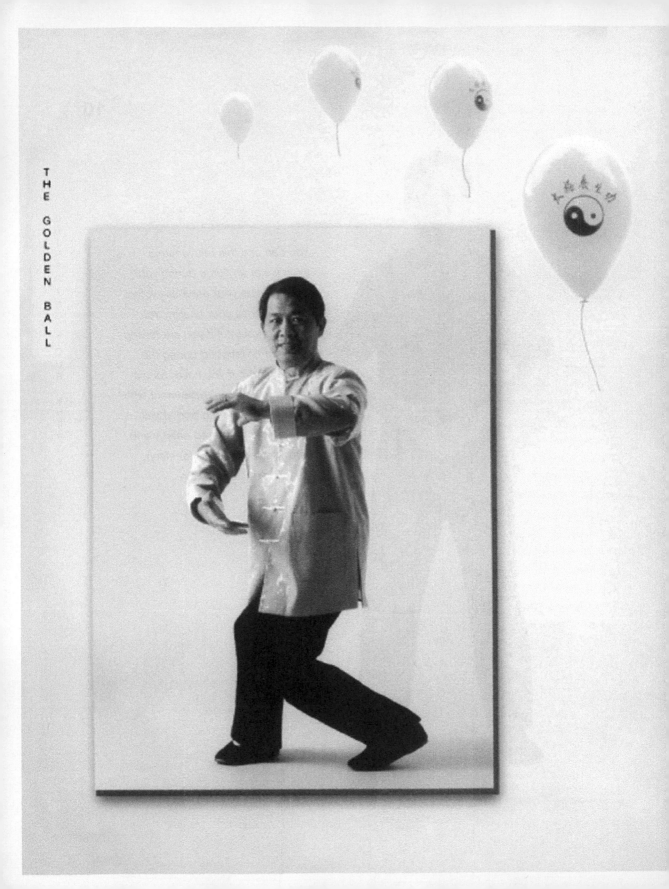

THE GOLDEN BALL

1 Shaking the ball

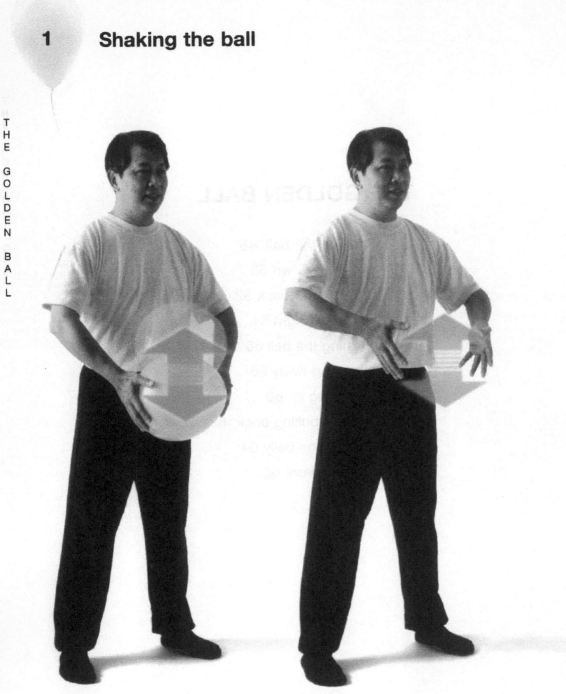

Imagine you are holding the large golden ball between your open palms in front of your belly.

It feels full and slightly heavy.

Your palms are slightly curved around the surface of the imaginary ball and your fingers are spread apart as if holding a large beach ball.

Shake the ball between your hands, making small quick movements, as if you were playing a shaker in the rhythm section of a band.

Keep your arms, elbows and hands relaxed. Do not hunch your shoulders or tighten the muscles in your upper arms.

The shaking motion does not need to be excessive: the imaginary ball moves only a few inches quickly up and down.

Breathe naturally.

Shake the golden ball for up to a minute.

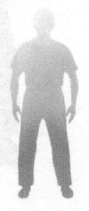

Return to Wu Chi

2　Up and down

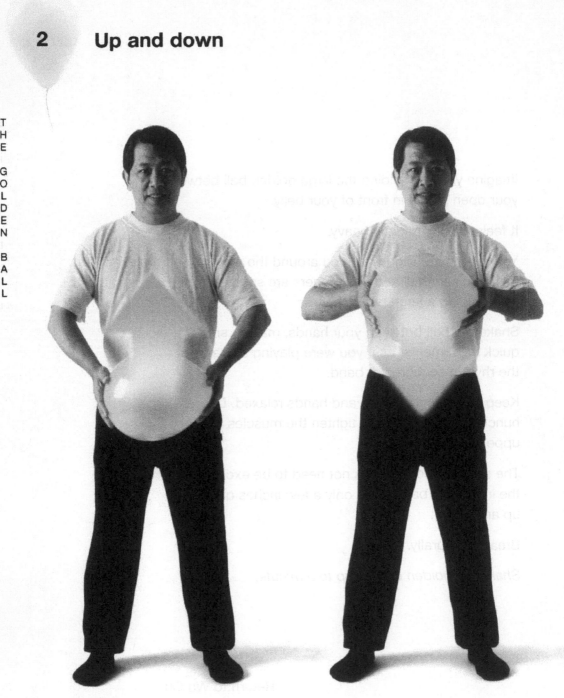

Hold the large golden ball between your palms in front of your belly. The ball fills the entire space between your palms.

Slowly lift the ball up until it is level with your chest. Breathe in as you raise the ball.

Then slowly lower the ball down to the starting position in front of your belly. Breathe out as you do this.

Imagine the ball is heavy and you are trying to move it up and down in thick oil. Doing the exercise with this idea in mind changes the nature of the movement. Instead of being a quick light movement without any apparent purpose, the movement becomes slow, deliberate and powerful. It has internal power, which grows as you practise regularly.

Continue raising and lowering the golden ball for a minute or two.

Return to Wu Chi

3 Forward and back

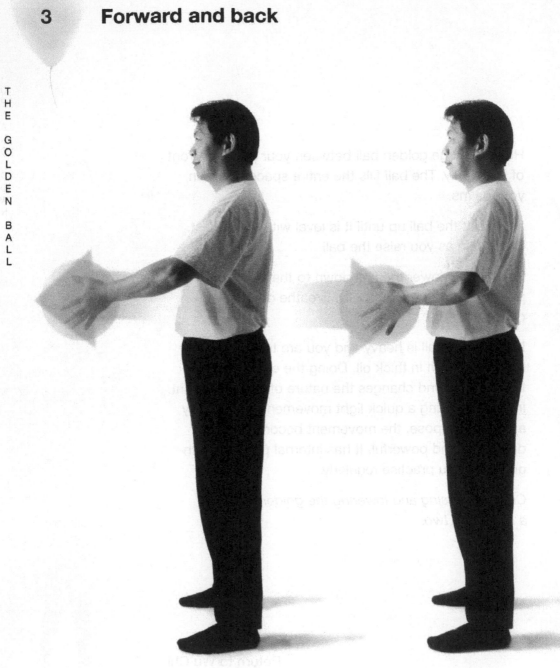

You hold the large golden ball between your palms in front of you. Your arms are slightly away from your body, with your shoulders and elbows relaxed.

Imagine your palms and fingers are completely in touch with the curved surface of the large ball. This ensures that your palms are gently curved and your fingers spread apart.

Slowly extend the ball away from you. Breathe out as you do this.

Be careful not to overextend your arms as you move the ball forward. Your elbows remain bent and you move the ball forward about ten to twelve inches.

Keep your elbows and shoulders relaxed.

Slowly move the ball back toward you. Breathe in as you do this.

Do not bring the ball in too close to your body. Try to keep the ball about six inches in front of you.

Imagine the air around the ball is dense, so that your movements are slow and thoughtful.

Practise moving the golden ball forward and back for a minute or two.

Return to Wu Chi

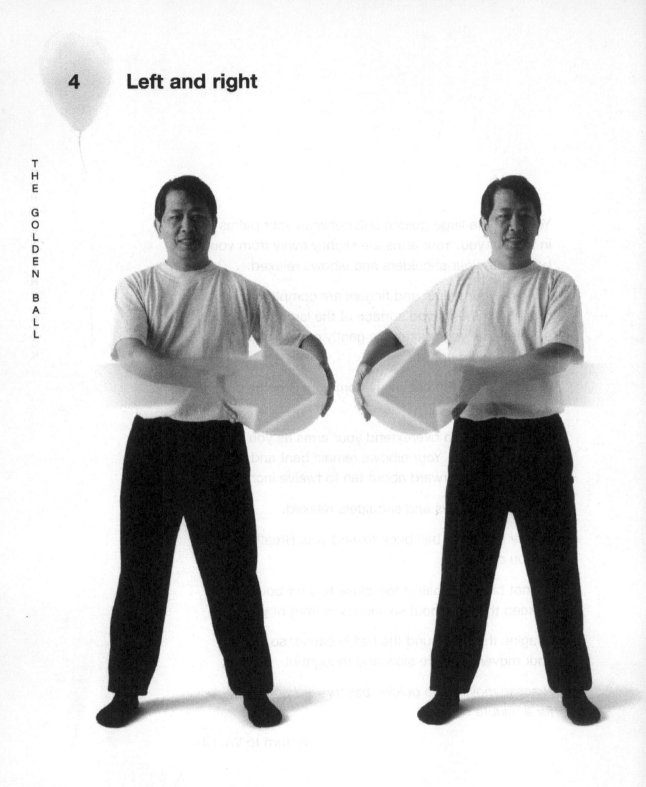

4 Left and right

Hold the large golden ball between your palms in front of you. Imagine the ball is half-filled with water. This makes it feel heavy, but not stiff. You feel that the space between your hands is filled with strong lively energy.

Slowly move the ball to the left without turning your body. Hold for a second.

Slowly bring it back to the centre. Hold for a second.

Then repeat the movement to the right.

Breathe naturally.

Without the imaginary ball between your hands, this movement feels empty and pointless. But if you use the power of your imagination to feel the heavy swaying motion of the water inside the ball as you move it, you will discover a hidden power within the movements of your hands and arms.

Practise this movement from left to right slowly for a minute or two.

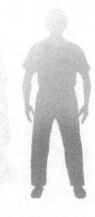

Return to Wu Chi

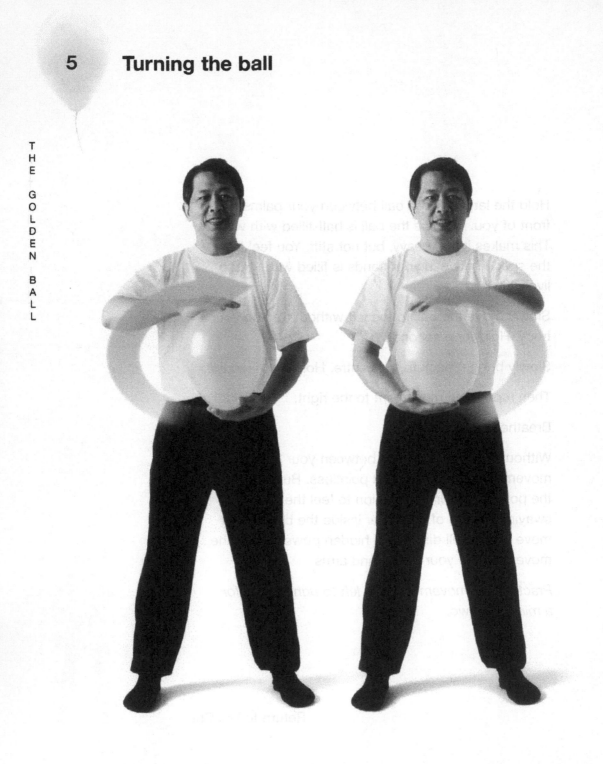

5 **Turning the ball**

Begin by holding the large golden ball in front of your belly. Relax your shoulders and chest, and rest in that position. Then slowly raise the ball until you are holding it in front of your chest.

Turn the ball so that your right hand is on top. Your left hand is cupped underneath. Hold the ball still for a few moments.

Then reverse the movement. Turn the ball over so that your left hand is on top and your right hand underneath. Hold the ball still for a moment or two.

Then turn the ball all the way back. Keep turning it over and back again without pausing. Develop a smooth rhythm, not too fast, not too slow.

Make sure your shoulders and elbows remain relaxed throughout the movement. Leave lots of space under your arms as you turn the ball.

Breathe naturally.

After turning the ball over a dozen times, hold the ball still with your right hand on top and left hand underneath. Then make another dozen or more turns, again pausing at the end with one hand on top and the other underneath.

Return to Wu Chi

6 **Sending away**

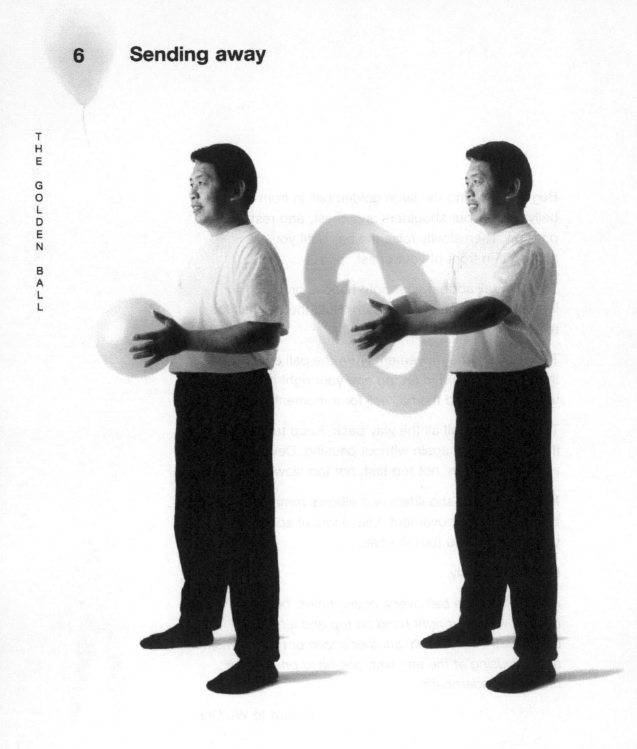

The large golden ball is between your palms. You are holding it just in front of your waist. Stand still for a moment before beginning this next movement.

Slowly move the golden ball up and away from your chest. It moves outward in a gentle curve, as if you were tracing the top curve of a large circle in front of you. Complete the circle by bringing the ball down and in towards your belly.

Keep your elbows loosely bent so that they move naturally with the movement of your hands.

Breathe out as the large ball circles up and outward. Breathe in as the ball comes down and in toward your belly.

This motion feels steady and full. As you move the ball through the space in front of you, it feels strong and heavy.

As you roll the ball away from you and breathe out, imagine your energy is sending away your aches and pains or any other problems in your life.

Make at least a dozen circles with the golden ball if you can.

Return to Wu Chi

7   Taking in

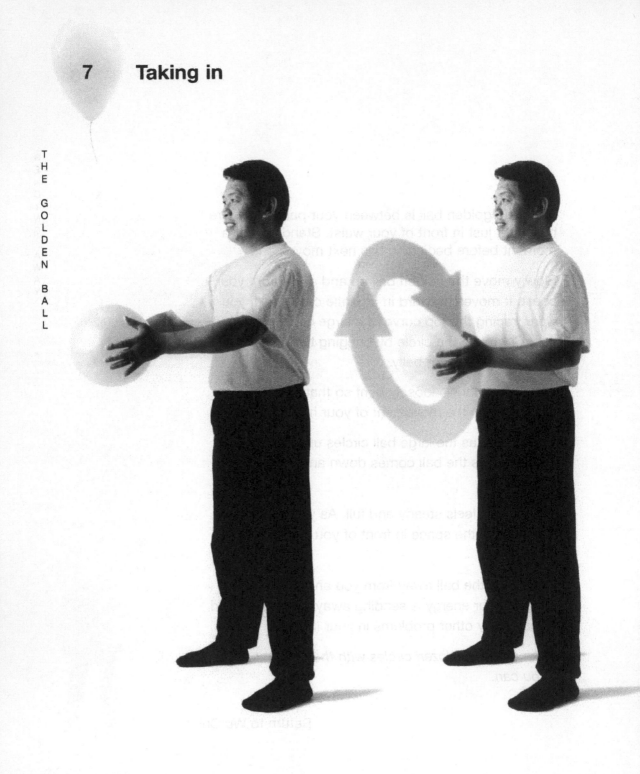

Stand still with the large golden ball between your
hands. Hold the imaginary ball a comfortable distance
away from your body.

Slowly start to move the ball in toward your chest.
As it comes toward you, let the ball curve down past
your chest and toward your belly.

Breathe in as the ball circles in toward you.

Keep your elbows loosely bent so that they move
naturally with the movement of your hands.

Complete the circle by bringing the ball up and out
in front of you.

Breathe out as the ball comes up and away from
your belly.

As you roll the golden ball toward you and breathe in,
feel you are taking positive energy in from the space
and light around you and nourishing the field of your
own energy.

*Make at least a dozen circles with the golden ball
if you can.*

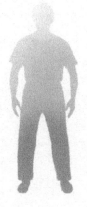

Return to Wu Chi

8   Pushing out, pulling back

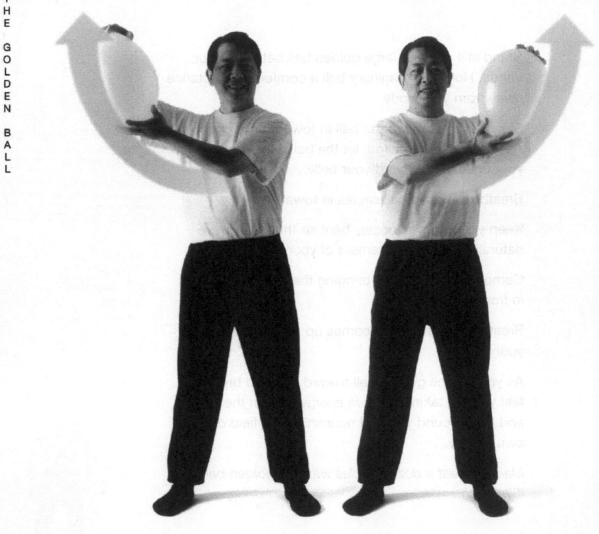

Hold the large golden ball between your palms in front of your chest.

Breathe in.

Move the ball out from in front of your chest to the upper right diagonal. Breathe out as you do this.

Now bring the ball back to your chest. Breathe in as you do this.

Then move the ball out from your chest up to the upper left diagonal. Breathe out as you do this.

Finish by bringing the ball back down again to your chest.

Complete this movement to both sides, 12 times.

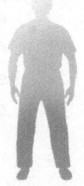

Return to Wu Chi

Holding the belly

The ancient Chinese art of internal exercise cultivates your entire energy field. You practise relaxing while holding an imaginary golden ball. As you hold the position, your energy circulates naturally around your body.

You increase your vitality by strengthening the complete field of your body's energy. This is the life-giving energy that circulates inside you, and also around you, at all times.

Completely relax your belly so that it expands naturally outward.

Bring both your hands up in front of your belly.

Imagine you are holding a large golden ball slightly away from your body, in front of your belly.

As you do this, relax your palms. Feel they are resting on the smooth curve of the golden ball.

Relax your shoulders.

Breathe naturally.

Gently hold the golden ball for a minute or two.

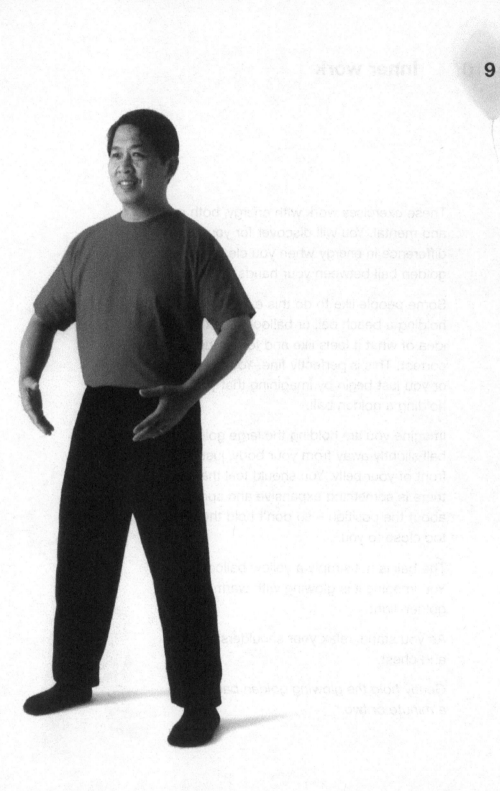

10 Inner work

These exercises work with energy, both physical and mental. You will discover for yourself the difference in energy when you clearly imagine the golden ball between your hands.

Some people like to do this exercise while actually holding a beach ball or balloon, just to get a clear idea of what it feels like and to get the position correct. This is perfectly fine. You can start this way, or you just begin by imagining that you are holding a golden ball.

Imagine you are holding the large golden ball slightly away from your body, just in front of your belly. You should feel that there is something expansive and spacious about the position – so don't hold the ball too close to you.

The ball is not simply a yellow balloon. You imagine it is glowing with warm golden light.

As you stand, relax your shoulders and chest.

Gently hold the glowing golden ball for a minute or two.

When holding this position, some people tend to hunch their shoulders and to strain their chest muscles as they hold their arms in front. One way to release that tension is to imagine that there is a strap running behind your neck and stretching down to your wrists. The strap takes all the weight of your arms and, at the same time, has the effect of lowering your shoulders and relaxing your chest.

Breathe naturally.

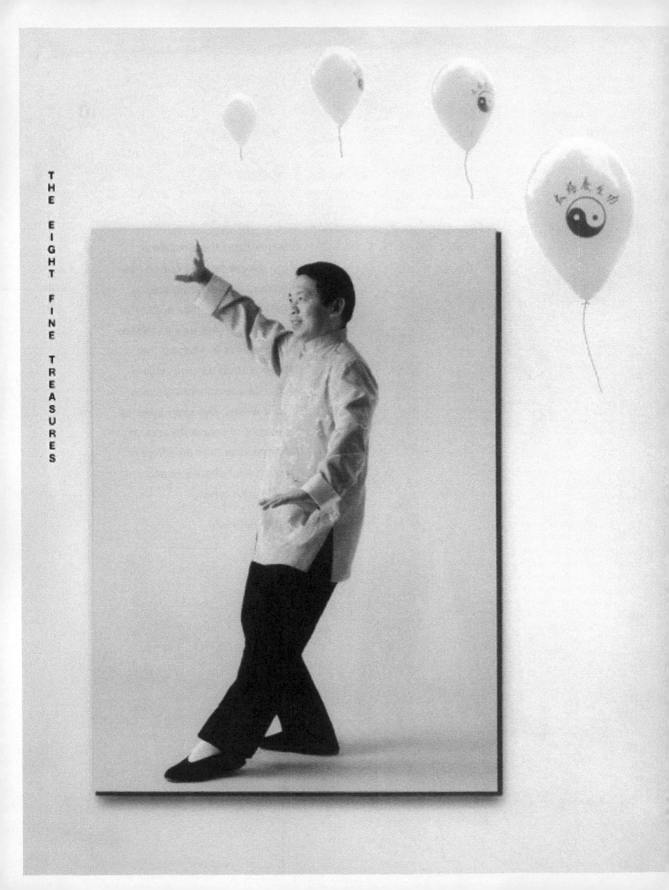

THE EIGHT FINE TREASURES

1 **Extending outward**

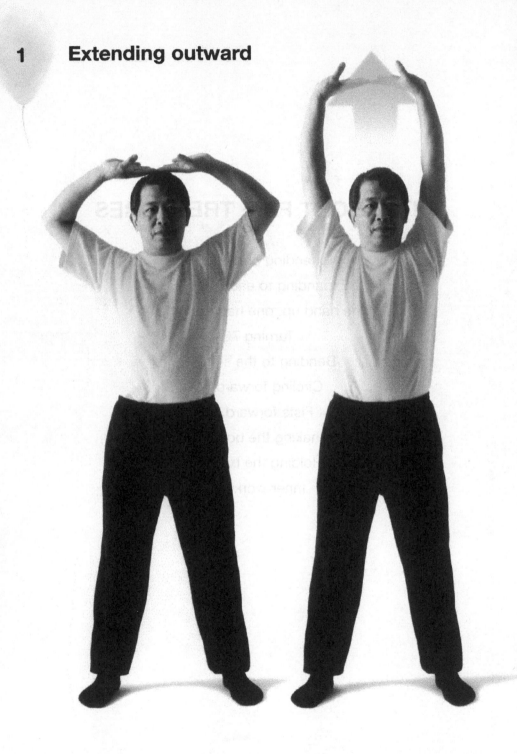

Stand with your feet shoulder width apart. Relax your shoulders and chest. Breathe out.

Raise your hands and turn your palms outward from your head or face.

Breathe in.

Slowly extend your arms, pressing your palms away from you. Breathe out as you do this.

Slowly bring your hands back to the starting position. Breathe in as you do this.

Extend outward like this, slowly and gently, eight times if you can.

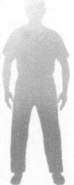

Return to Wu Chi

2 Expanding to each side

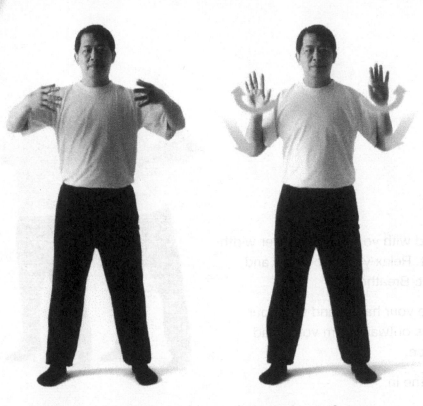

Raise your palms toward your chest, in front of your shoulders.

Turn your palms outward to each side. Breathe in.

Slowly expand, pressing each palm to the side.
Breathe out as you do this.

Slowly return your arms to the starting position.
Breathe in as you do this.

Breathe naturally and begin again.

Repeat this expansion, slowly and gently, eight times.

One hand up, one hand down

2

Imagine you are opening two large sliding doors. This makes your movement slow, deliberate and powerful.

Return to Wu Chi

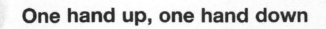

3 One hand up, one hand down

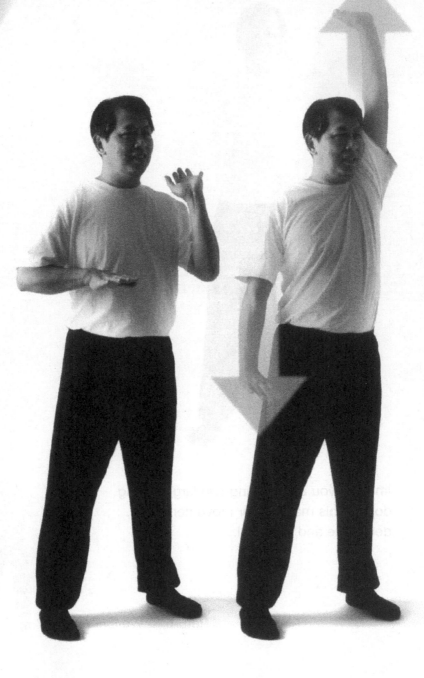

Stand with your feet shoulder width apart. Relax your neck, shoulders and chest.

Imagine you are holding a large inflated ball between your hands in front of your chest.

Breathe in.

Move one hand upward, so that the palm is facing the sky. Your hand is in position as if you were carrying a tray on it just above your shoulder. At the same time, move the other hand downward, so that the palm is facing the earth. This hand is in position as if you were resting your hand on top of a high stool level with your hips.

As you breathe out, extend both arms, pushing away with the palms, one up and one down. Try to keep both palms flat, at right angles to your forearms. As you do this, you feel a stretch in your wrists.

Hold the stretch for a second.

Breathe in as you bring both hands back in front of you, holding the invisible balloon.

Change hands and repeat the stretch. Make eight stretches if you can, alternating the hands.

Return to Wu Chi

4 Turning

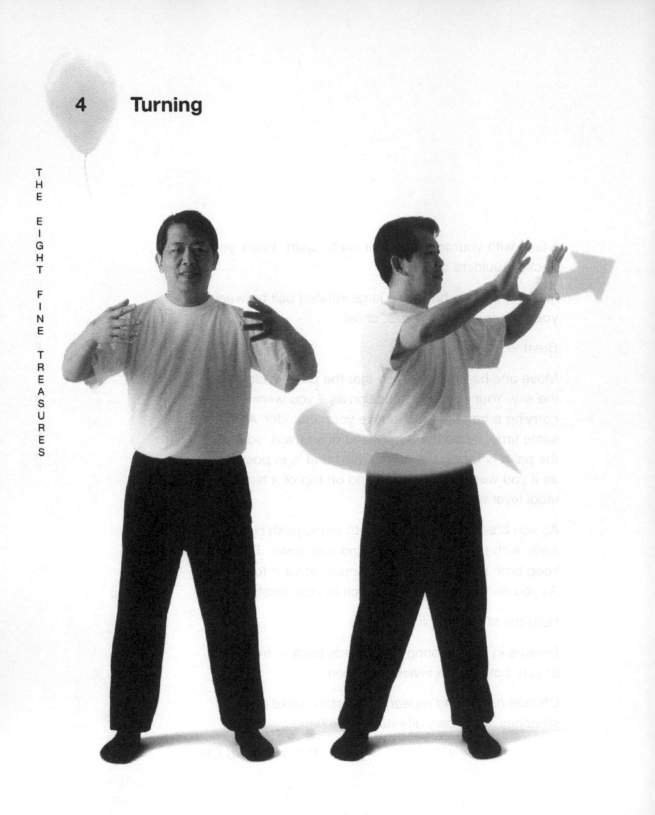

Stand with your feet shoulder width apart, feeling a strong connection between the ground and the soles of your feet.

Imagine you are holding a large inflated ball between your hands in front of your chest.

Breathe in.

Slowly turn your hips to the left. Your entire upper body moves with this turn. Open your palms outwards as you turn. Breathe out as you make this movement.

Keep your neck, chest and shoulders relaxed. Your hands feel slightly expanded with your fingers gently spread apart.

Hold for a second.

Slowly turn back to the front. Breathe in as you do this. You are again holding the imaginary ball in front of your chest.

Make eight turns if you can, alternating to each side.

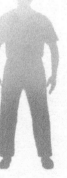

5 **Bending to the side**

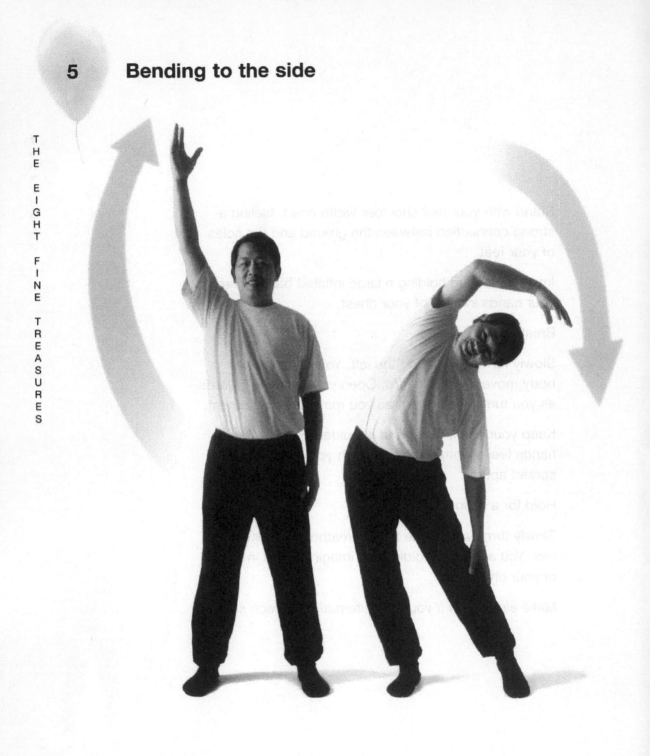

Stand with your feet shoulder width apart. Relax your neck, shoulders and chest.

Raise your right hand up over your head. If you find that difficult, rest your forearm on the top of your head so that your hand touches the tip of your left ear. Breathe in as you raise your arm into position.

Shift your weight to your right leg. Breathe out and feel your weight sinking firmly down onto your foot. To help this, try slightly raising your left heel, so that only the toes and ball of the left foot are on the ground.

Breathe in.

Lean over to your left side, so that you feel a gentle stretch along the right side of your body. Breathe out as you lean to the left. You can feel secure leaning over to the left a little because you have shifted your centre of gravity safely over to your right side. You can stabilize yourself as you bend by pressing a little on the ball of your left foot, if you need to.

Repeat this bending exercise eight times, alternating to each side.

6 Circling forward

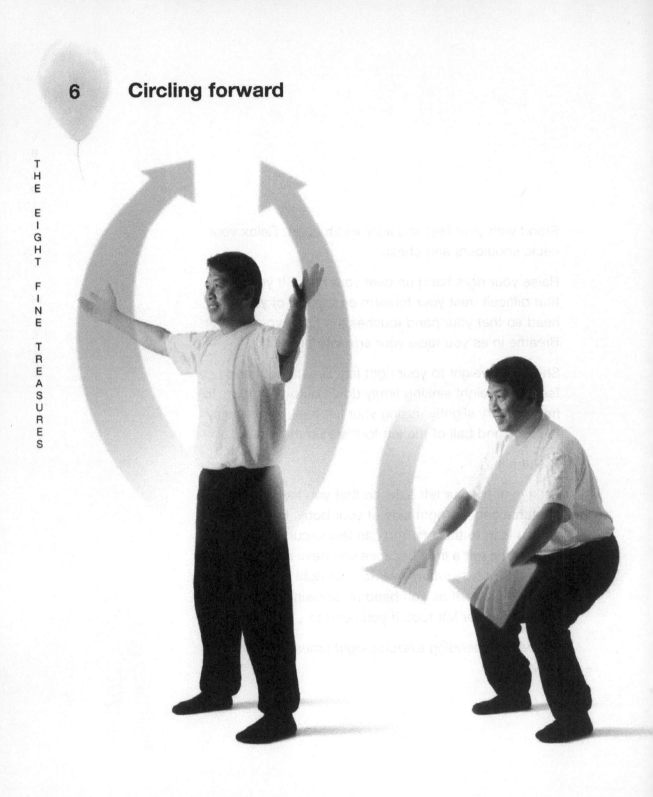

Stand with your feet shoulder width apart. Look forward. Relax your shoulders and chest.

Slowly raise your arms out to the sides and let them come up to shoulder height. Your palms face upward. Breathe in.

Circle your arms forward, bringing your hands out in front of your body with your palms facing downward. Your arms circle forward and down until they touch your knees. Lean forward and bend your knees a little so your hands can touch them.

Breathe out as you circle your arms forward and your knees bend.

Try not to drop your head too much, but don't keep it stiffly upright.

Straighten up, breathe naturally and get ready to repeat the movement.

Make eight complete forward circles with your arms if you can.

Return to Wu Chi

7 Fists forward

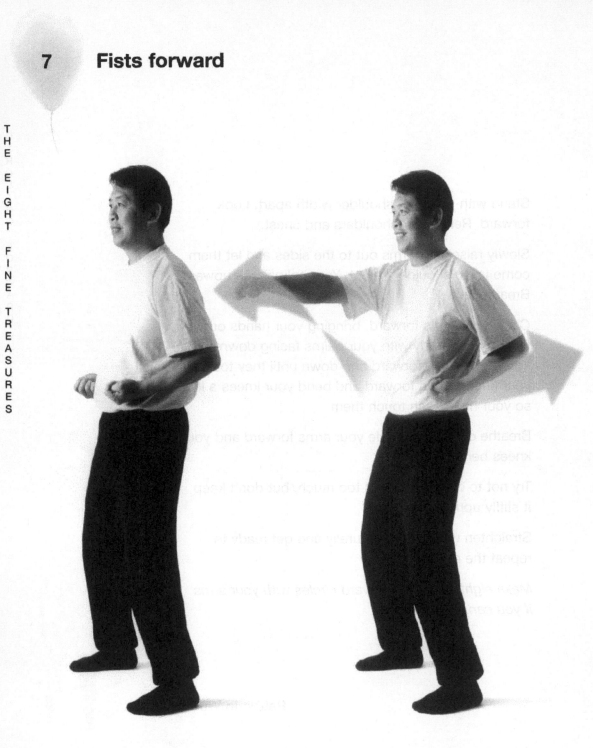

Stand with your feet shoulder width apart. Relax your upper body, letting your weight sink down through the soles of your feet.

Make fists with your thumbs inside your fingers. Hold them beside your hips with your palms facing upward.

Breathe in.

Slowly extend your right fist forward, turning it so that your palm now faces downward. At the same time, pull your left fist slightly backward beside your hip. Feel you are stretching a strong piece of elastic between your hands, and squeeze your thumbs inside your fists. Breathe out as you squeeze.

Relax the squeeze and bring your fists back beside your hips. Breathe in as you do this.

Now slowly extend your left fist forward, palm down. Pull your right fist backward, palm up. Feel the elastic being stretched between them. Breathe out as you extend and squeeze your thumbs.

Look straight ahead.

Make eight of these stretches if you can.

Return to Wu Chi

8 Shaking the body

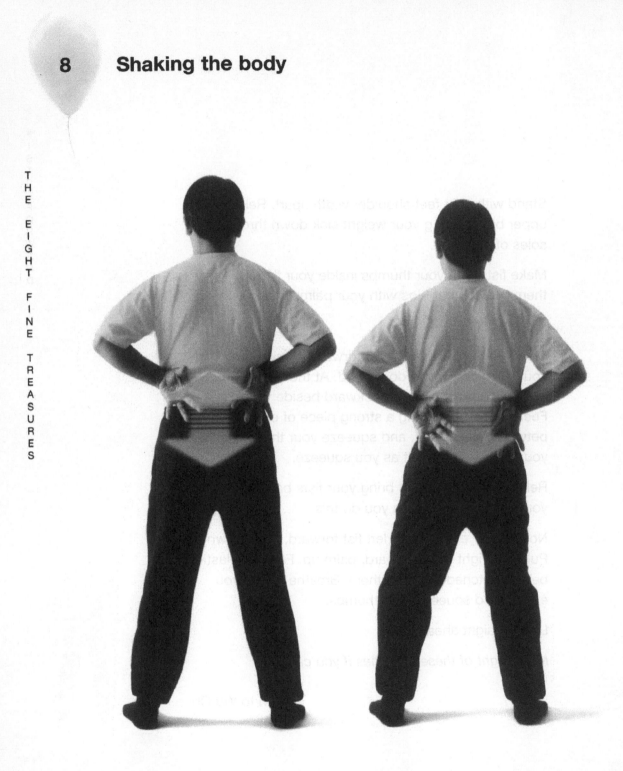

Stand with your feet shoulder width apart. Breathe naturally.

Rest the backs of your hands in the small of your back just above your hip bones. Relax your elbows and shoulders.

You feel as if you are resting the full weight of your arms on the backs of your wrists in the small of your back.

Breathe in.

Keeping your feet firmly on the floor, use your knees to bounce your body up and down, as if you were riding a horse. Your relaxed arms will respond naturally to the movement of your body so that the backs of your hands naturally massage the area around your kidneys. Breathe out as you shake.

Stop shaking, breathe in and prepare to repeat.

Shake yourself, giving your kidneys this relaxing massage, eight times if you can.

Return to Wu Chi

9   Holding the ball

Each time you hold the golden ball you are increasing the flow of your body's vital energy. The different positions have been handed down over the centuries by masters who studied the subtle movement of energy in the human body.

Holding the ball at the level of your chest relieves pressure on your internal organs, improves your breathing and boosts the circulation of blood and energy all the way to your feet, hands and brain.

Imagine you are holding a large golden ball slightly away from your body, in front of your belly. Your palms rest along its smooth curve.

Slowly let the ball rise up so that you hold it slightly away from your body in front of your chest.

Check that you have not raised your shoulders when raising your arms. Let your shoulders relax and sink down.

Make sure there is space under your armpits. This avoids your arms pressing against your ribcage, allowing your lungs more freedom as you breathe.

Let your breathing be completely natural.

9

As you can see from the photo of Master Lam, lower yourself about an inch as if you were just starting to sit down.

Gently rest in position, holding the golden ball at chest level, with your arms comfortably sinking into the two balloons floating on the water in front of you.

Begin with a couple of minutes if you can manage that. Then increase, day by day, until you find that you can stand for between 5 and 15 minutes, inwardly relaxed and still.

10 Inner work

This position is more powerful than the earlier posture of Holding the belly (pages 64–67). It is therefore all the more important to do the accompanying inner work of relaxation.

In order to support yourself properly when you dip down at the hips, imagine that you are starting to sit on a very large imaginary ball – like a huge exercise ball – that is placed below you on the floor. You literally imagine that you are sinking your weight down on this large ball, just as if it was there. The feeling is similar to resting your backside on a high stool.

To relax your shoulders and elbows, imagine you are holding the large golden ball so that it is lightly held between your chest, forearms and hands. Your palms rest along its smooth curve.

Imagine your arms are supported by balloons under your armpits and forearms. As you stand, you will find that you can feel the weight of your arms sinking into these balloons. You will find that you need to use far less muscle power to hold your arms in position – they remain in place, naturally relaxed.

Breathe naturally.

Gently rest in that position with the golden ball in your arms for a minute or two.

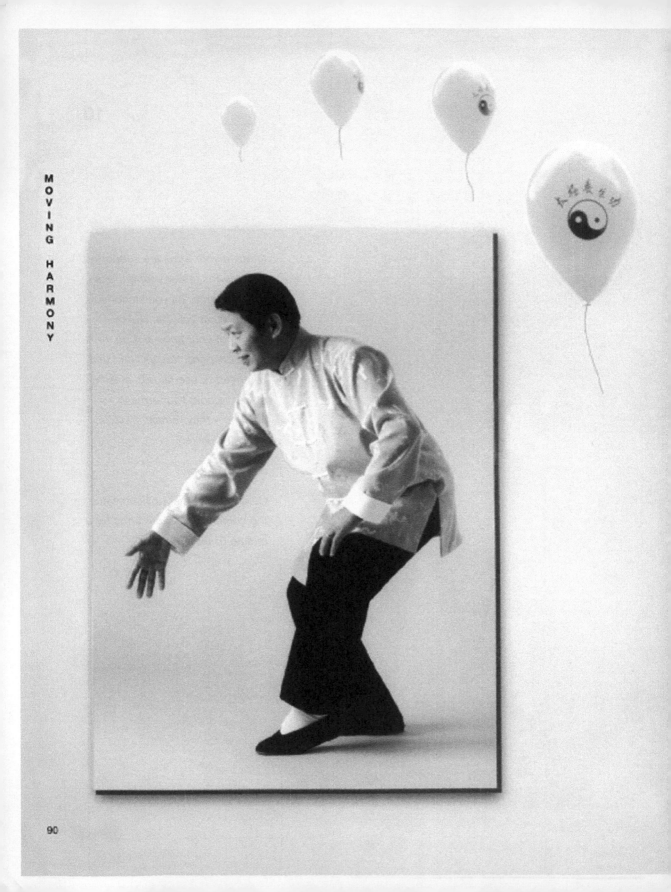

MOVING HARMONY

1   Forward pushing

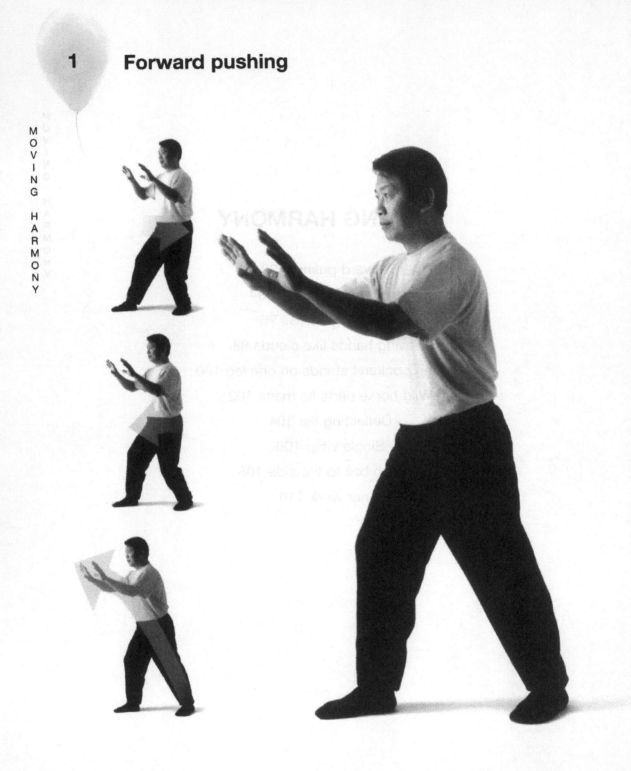

Stand with your feet shoulder width apart. Turn your left foot diagonally outward. Step forward with your right foot.

Sink most of your weight onto your left foot. Both your knees are slightly bent.

Raise your arms in front of your chest with your palms facing forward, as if you were about to push on a large, heavy door with both hands.

Breathe in.

Press against the door, powering the push with your rear leg until you have transferred your weight forward and slightly extended your arms.

Breathe out as you push forward. Be careful not to straighten your arms or lean forward over your toes.

Relax, return to the starting posture, breathing in.

Repeat this movement eight times. Then repeat it eight times with your feet in the opposite position – left foot forward, right foot back.

Return to Wu Chi

2   Single hand pushing

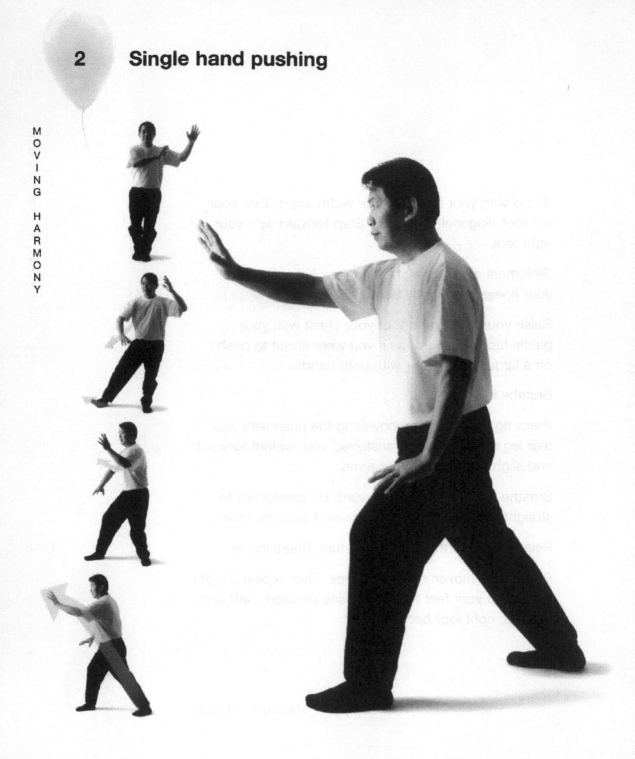

Stand with your feet together. Rest your weight fully on your left foot, and lift your right heel slightly. Bend your knees a little. Raise your left hand out to the side, bring your right palm up across your chest to rest in front of your left shoulder.

Swing your right leg outward bringing your heel to rest on the ground, with your foot pointing out to the side. At the same time lower your right hand down beside your hip.

Slowly shift your weight onto your right foot, turning your torso toward the right and pushing your left hand forward. At the same time, swivel on your left foot so that both your feet end up pointing in the same direction.

Repeat the movement to the other side, starting with your weight on your right foot and extending your left foot to the side.

Try to complete six of the movements to each side.

Return to Wu Chi

3   **Sweeping across**

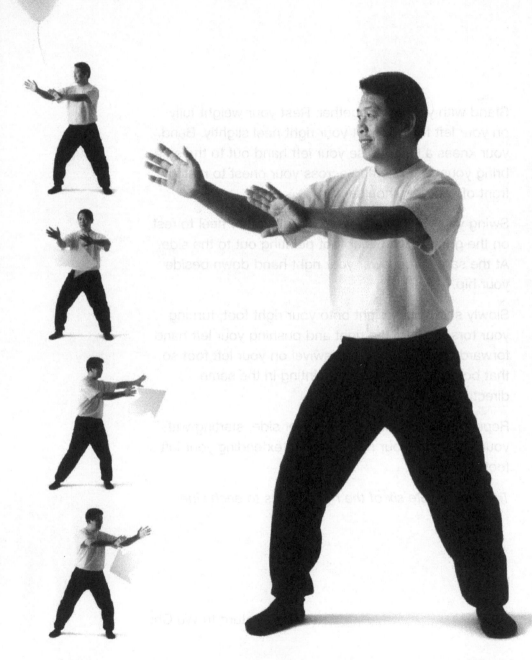

Stand with your feet a little wider apart than shoulder width. Sit down slightly so that both knees are bent, keeping your back upright. Raise both arms out to the right side, with your palms turned to face forward. Your hands are level with your shoulders.

Turn your hips toward the left, allowing your torso and arms to move with the turn.

Complete the sweep by letting your right knee follow the movement until you are turned toward the left as far as possible without discomfort. The amount of turn will vary from person to person.

Once you have turned to the left side, swivel your hands to face forward and prepare to sweep back across to the right.

Sweep across eight times, alternating from side to side.

Return to Wu Chi

MOVING HARMONY

4 Waving hands like clouds

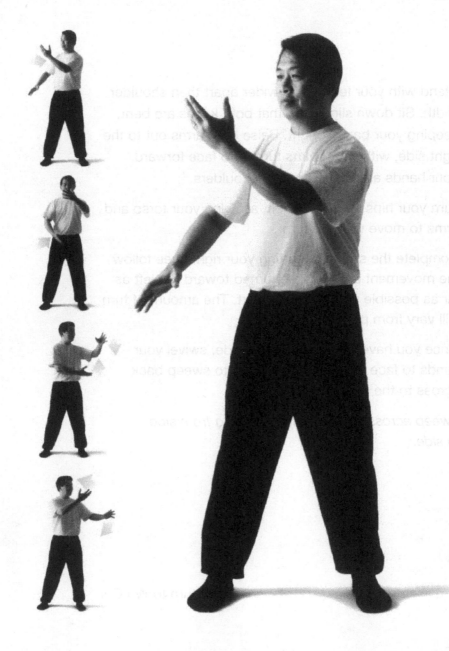

Stand with your feet shoulder width apart. Relax your chest and shoulders. Hold your left hand facing you in front of your chest, your fingers slightly spread. Hold your right hand away from your body at waist level, palm downward, fingers spread.

Slowly move your left hand up in front of you, turning from the hips toward the left. Your whole torso moves with the turn.

Continue the movement of your left hand to make a large outward circle to the side, as you complete turning to that side. As your left hand moves upward and outward, your right hand also circles up, preparing to make a large curve outward to the right.

Having turned to the left, you slowly turn to the right. Your right hand leads the movement, circling outward to the right. As you do this, your left hand slowly starts to come up in front of you, in preparation for your next turn to the left.

Your head turns with the movement of the body, watching your hands moving by like clouds.

Make eight complete slow turns of the body.

Return to Wu Chi

5 Golden cockerel stands on one leg

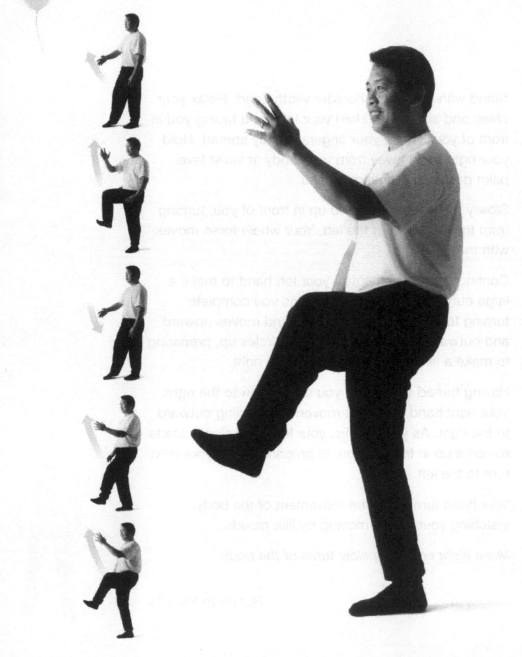

GOLDEN COCKEREL STANDS ON ONE LEG

Begin by standing upright with your heels together and your toes pointing slightly outward, forming a 45 degree angle. Hold your hands loosely in front of you near your hips.

Transfer your weight onto your left foot. Raise your right knee as high as you can without losing your balance. At the same time, raise your right hand to shoulder height. It may be helpful to imagine an invisible thread connecting your hand with your knee. If you are unstable, you can practise this using the wall or a chair for support.

Raise and lower your legs and arms eight times, alternating to each side if you are able.

If you are using a support, raise your right arm and leg four times and then your left arm and leg four times.

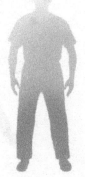

Return to Wu Chi

6 Wild horse parts its mane

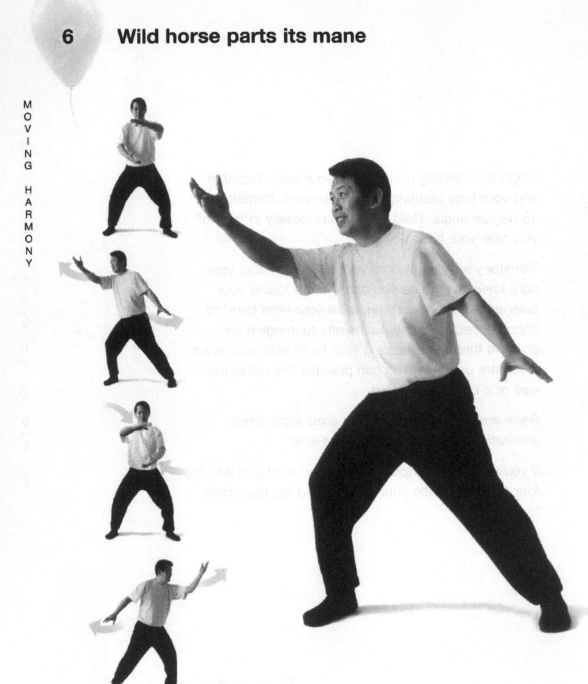

This movement takes its name from the energy of
a powerful horse tossing its head from side to side,
its mane flying in the wind.

Spread your feet slightly wider than shoulder width.
Lower yourself a couple of inches.

Hold the large imaginary ball between your hands.
Your left hand is on top, your right hand below.

Slice your right hand outwards to the upper right
diagonal, above and beyond your right shoulder.
At the same time, slice your left hand down to the
lower left diagonal, below and beyond your left hip,
shifting your weight to the right side.

Shift your weight back to the centre, bringing both
arms in to hold the ball in front of you. Now your
right hand is on top, your left hand below.

Repeat the movement to the other side. Your left
hand moves up the upper diagonal; your right hand
swings downward.

Breathe out as your arms slice out, breathe in as
you return to holding the golden ball.

Repeat the movement to both sides 12 times.

Return to Wu Chi

7 Deflecting fist

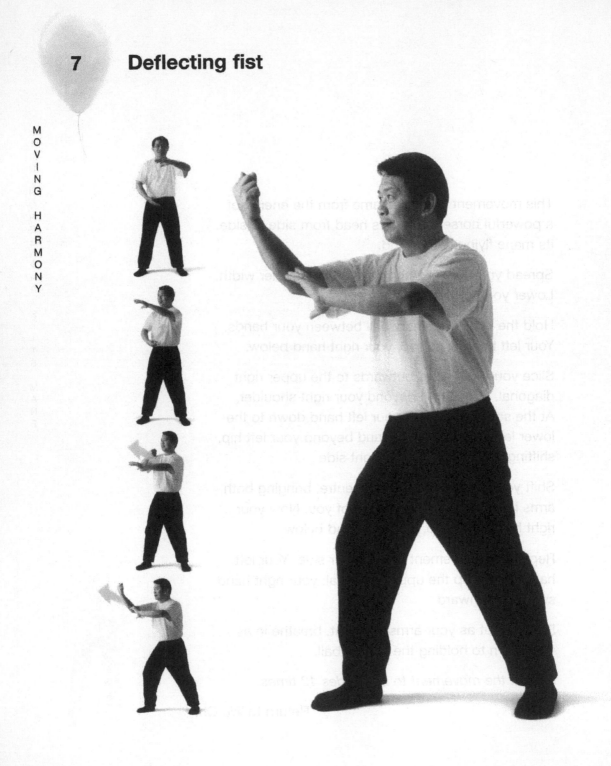

Stand with your feet shoulder width apart. Imagine you are holding a large ball between your hands, right hand underneath, left hand on top.

Fold your right hand into a loose fist and turn your hips slightly to the right.

Circle your right fist up until it is in front of your neck, slightly higher than your left hand, which moves slightly downward.

Transfer your weight forward onto your right foot and move your forearm forward. Be careful not to lean forward over your toes.

Repeat the movement, four times to the right and four times to the left.

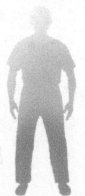

Return to Wu Chi

8   Single whip

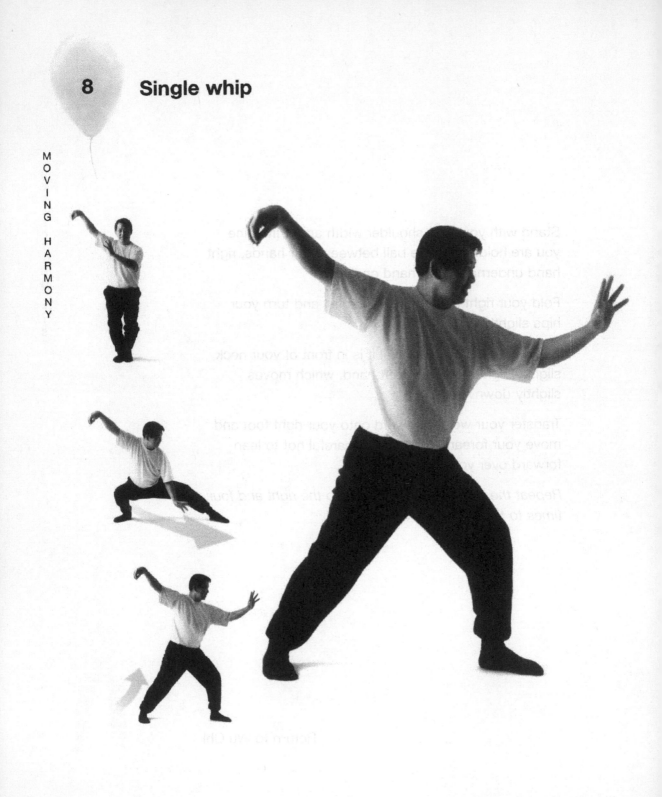

This is a demanding movement which should not be attempted until you are fully confident with all of the other movements. You will probably have difficulty sinking as low as Master Lam demonstrates here. Sink down only as far as is comfortable, it does not matter if this is just a few inches.

Start with your feet together, all your weight on your right foot. Lift your left heel slightly off the ground.

Make a downward "hook" with your right hand by gently squeezing the pads of your fingertips against the pad of your thumb tip. Extend the "hook" outward and upward to the right. Bring your left hand across your chest in front of your right shoulder.

Swing your left foot outward to the side, and lower your left hand to waist height.

Drop slowly down, keeping your weight on your right foot, and allowing your left foot to slide forward as far as is comfortable.

Shift your weight completely over to your left foot and slowly rise, straightening your right leg and pulling it in, while extending your left arm forward.

Repeat the movement eight times, alternating to the left and right.

Return to Wu Chi

9   **Golden ball to the side**

This is the most powerful of the Chi Kung positions you are introduced to in this book. It raises your inner power to much higher levels. For this reason, it should only be practised after you have completed learning all the previous positions and movements.

To begin, stand in the Wu Chi position with your feet shoulder width apart. Relax your shoulders.

Then raise your arms to hold the large imaginary ball in front of your chest. Remain in that position for a minute, sinking your weight into imaginary balloons under your armpits and forearms (pages 86–89).

Turn your right foot on the heel to point to the right. Your feet are now at right angles. Your body turns naturally toward the right, as you turn your foot.

Rest 60 per cent of your weight on your left leg, allowing yourself to sink down over that leg as if resting your left buttock on a high stool.

Imagine the balloon between your hands is inflating slightly, causing your right hand to expand outwards.

Gradually build up to holding this position for a minute or two, first turning to the right and then to the left.

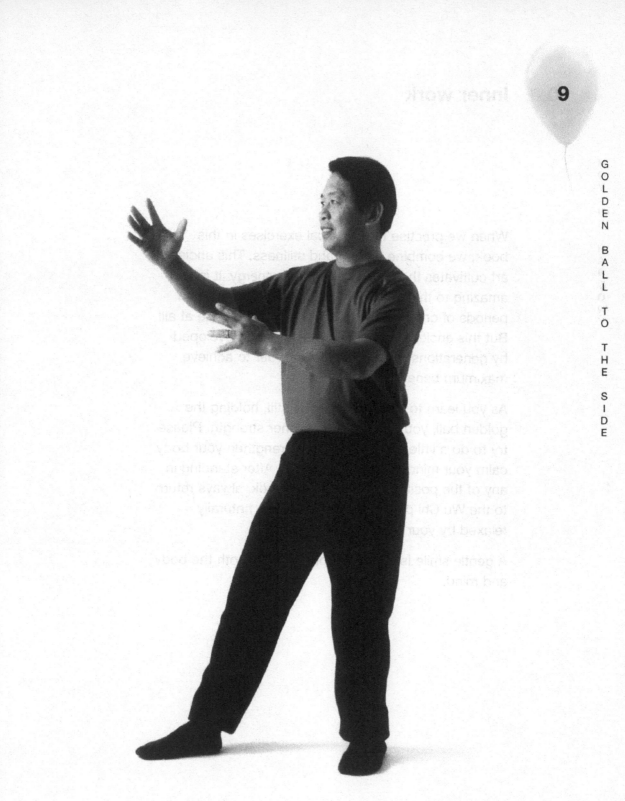

10   Inner work

When we practise the classical exercises in this book, we combine motion and stillness. This ancient art cultivates the entire field of your energy. It is amazing to think that such gentle movements, and periods of complete stillness, could be exercise at all! But this ancient art has been tested and developed by generations of practitioners in order to achieve maximum benefit.

As you learn to stand completely still, holding the golden ball, you can feel a new inner strength. Please try to do a little every day. It will strengthen your body, calm your mind and lift your spirits. After standing in any of the positions shown in this book, always return to the Wu Chi position, with your arms naturally relaxed by your sides.

A gentle smile is always helpful to relax both the body and mind.

"Your mind must be in your postures since it controls the use and direction of your power. At the same time you could smile: this is the inner laughter. That inner happiness will continue throughout your whole life.

The more you stand, the more comfortable you feel. Everything looks very soft, relaxed and at ease. Yet there is immense power inside you which, when channelled by the mind, expresses itself in movement."

MADAME WANG YUK-FONG, DAUGHTER OF GRAND MASTER WANG XIANG-ZHAI.

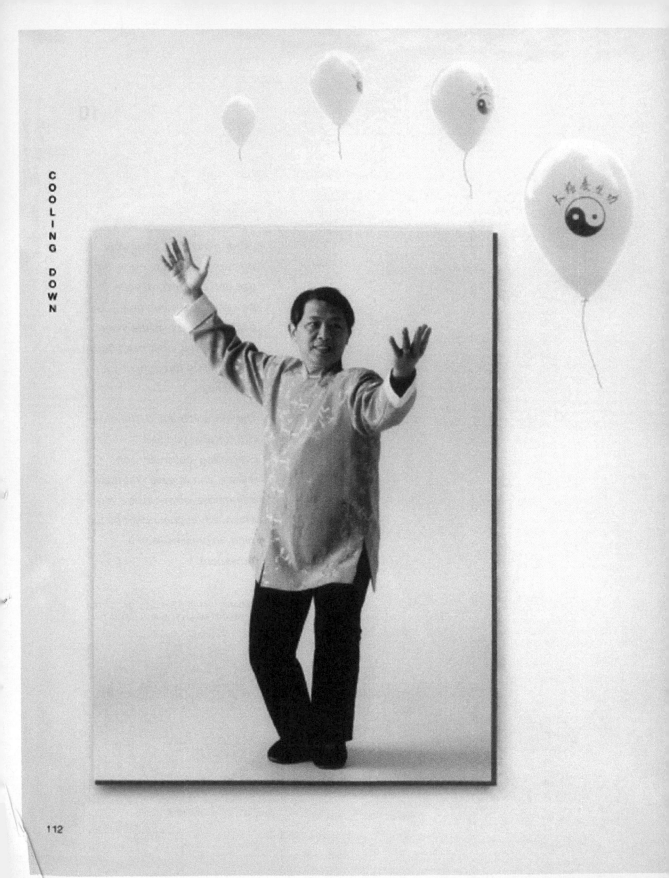

COOLING DOWN

1 Front and back

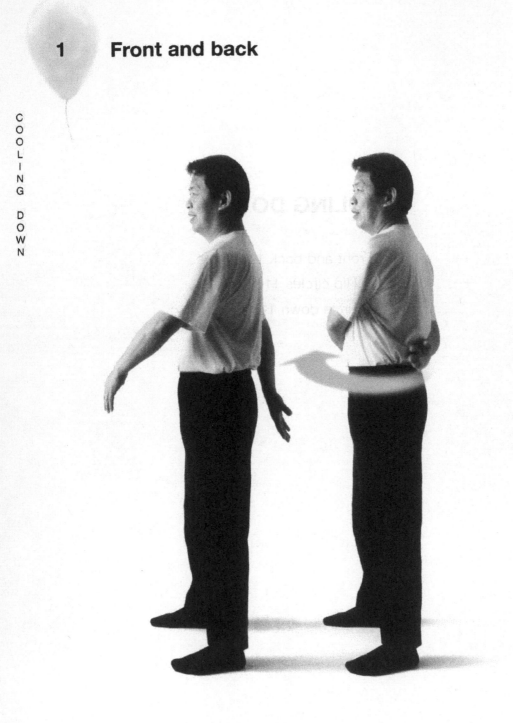

When you have finished your main training of the day, it is essential to cool down. The three exercises shown on the following pages help to release any tension that might have built up during your training and ensure that the energy you have generated is properly stored in your body.

This first cool down exercise helps release tension in your upper body and strengthens the energy in your abdomen and lower back.

Stand with your feet shoulder width apart to stabilize yourself for a moment.

Swing your left forearm in front of your body so that it bounces against your abdomen. At the same time swing your right forearm around behind your back so that it bounces against your lower back.

You feel the wrist of your front forearm bouncing on your belly below your navel. The wrist of your rear arm bounces on the midpoint of your lower back.

Then the swing reverses, so that your right arm comes in front and your left arm swings behind you. Let your shoulders and elbows be as relaxed as possible while you swing.

Breathe naturally.

Repeat this movement until you have completed up to 12 swings.

Return to Wu Chi

2 Hip circles

116

This cool down relaxes the hips and abdomen and releases tension in the major joints of the lower body. It should be done calmly and slowly, as if you were rolling a large stone ball.

Stand with your feet shoulder width apart. Rest your hands on your hips. Let your shoulders and elbows sink down.

Slowly move your hips in a large circle, starting in a clockwise direction – your hips move first forward to the right.

As you make the full circle with your hips, imagine your head is suspended by a fine cord. This keeps your head upright while your hips move.

Your knees should be straight (but not tightly locked).

Continue to keep your head up and your knees straight.

Breathe naturally.

Circle clockwise eight times. Then make eight large circles in the opposite direction, moving anti-clockwise.

Return to Wu Chi

3   Circle down

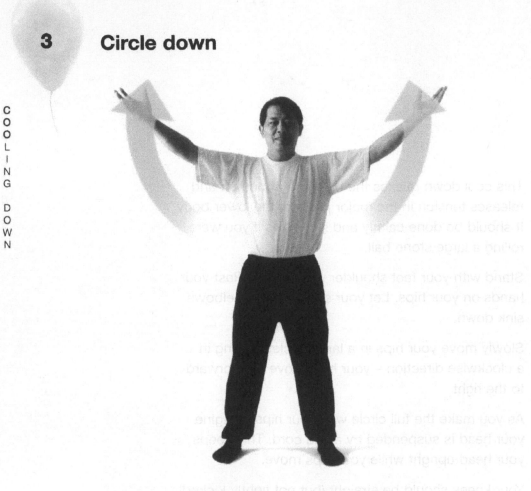

This final movement directs your energy into your abdomen, the natural reservoir of our vital energy, and seals it there. You should always conclude your daily exercise with this practice.

Raise both arms up beside your body in two large circles until your hands start to come toward each other above your head, slightly away from the front line of your body.

Breathe in as your arms circle up.

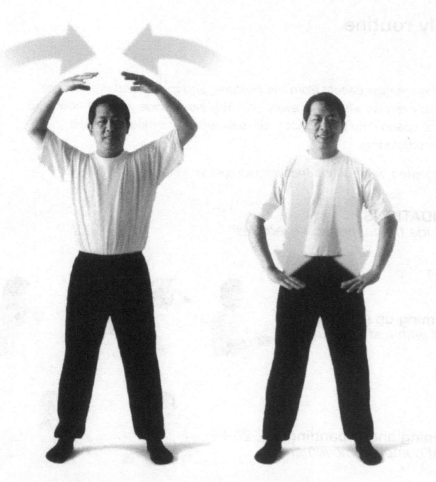

Then slowly press your hands down in front of you, feeling you are pressing a large ball down into water. The movement continues until your palms have pressed down in front of your belly. Breathe out as your arms press down.

Make three large circles, slowly and calmly. Then, slowly and calmly, fold your hands over your abdomen. Your right hand is against your belly, your left hand over it. Rest in stillness, breathing naturally for thirty seconds to a minute.

Return to Wu Chi

Your daily routine

You will get the greatest benefit from the postures and movement in this book if you do a little exercise with them every day. You can decide yourself how long you are able to spend. You can adapt your daily routine to meet your own needs and circumstances.

Here is a suggested daily routine that will help get you started:

THE FOUNDATIONS
Always include the foundation exercises

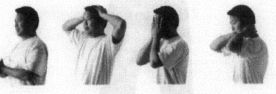

Warming up (pp. 26–27)
Start with half a minute

Opening and expanding (pp. 28–29)
Eight complete movements

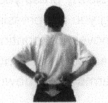

Standing and knuckling (pp. 30–31)
Up to a minute

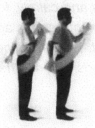

Swinging the forearms (pp. 32–33)
At least thirty swings

Shaking the body (pp. 34–35)
Up to a minute

Swimming on land (pp. 36–37)
Eight complete strokes

Standing in Wu Chi (pp. 38–39)
Begin with a minute or two

Standing and opening (pp. 40–43)
Continue in position for a minute or two

Gathering your energy (pp. 44–45)
Complete The Foundations with a minute or two

THE GOLDEN BALL

Shaking the ball (pp. 48–49)
Up to a minute

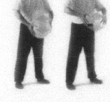

Up and down (pp. 50–51)
A minute or two

Forward and back (pp. 52–53)
A minute or two

Left and right (pp. 54–55)
A minute or two

Turning the ball (pp. 56–57)
Twelve times in each position

Sending away (pp. 58–59)
At least twelve circles

Taking in (pp. 60–61)
At least twelve circles

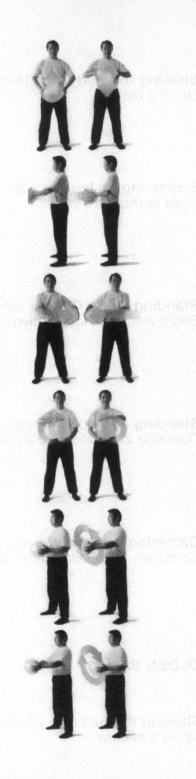

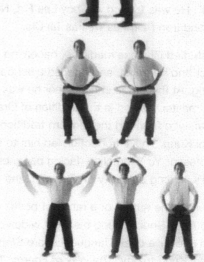

Pushing out, pulling back (pp. 62–63)
Complete movement twelve times

Holding the belly (pp. 64–65)
A minute or two

COOLING DOWN
Always finish with the Cooling Down movements

Front and back (pp. 114–115)
Twelve swings

Hip circles (pp. 116–117)
Eight times in each direction

Circle down (pp. 118–119)
Three circles

*When you are comfortable with this routine you can start to add in movements
from The Eight Fine Treasures, after The Golden Ball movements.
After several months' practice you can move on to including the Moving
Harmony movements, either after The Eight Fine Treasures (if you have time) or
instead of them from time to time.*

Master Lam Kam-Chuen

Master Lam has helped millions on the road to health. He has devoted his life to the study of Tai Chi and the healing arts of Chinese culture. From an early age he learned under some of the greatest masters of his time in Hong Kong, Taiwan and China. He has been teaching in the West since 1975, opening up the secrets of Chinese health care through his books, videos, workshops and classes. He was the first teacher appointed to lead Tai Chi classes in the Inner London Education Authority, opening the way for the hundreds of such classes now provided to people of all ages throughout the country.

Master Lam first studied under masters such as Leung Tse-Cheung (facing page, bottom left and right), a disciple of Grand Master Ku Yue-Chang, known throughout China as "the king of Iron Palm". He was trained in Choy Lee Fut, Northern Shaolin Kung Fu and Iron Palm, as well as Tai Chi.

He then studied Chinese medicine, becoming a qualified bonesetter and herbalist, and opened a school and clinic in Hong Kong. At this stage in his career he was introduced to a Chi Kung master, trained in the tradition of Grand Master Wang Xiang-Zhai, who founded the modern tradition of Da Cheng Chuan Chi Kung. This introduction led him to study in Beijing under Professor Yu Yong-Nian (facing page, bottom centre), now the world's leading authority on Zhan Zhuang Chi Kung.

Master Lam is the author of a range of books on Tai Chi, Chi Kung and Feng Shui. Among his most widely read works, published in over a dozen languages, are *Step-by-step Tai Chi* and his Chi Kung trilogy: *The Way of Energy, The Way of Healing* and *The Way of Power*. Television viewers will be familiar with Master Lam as the presenter of the 10-part Channel 4 series, *Stand Still – Be Fit,* now released as a Channel 4 video.

Facing page: *Tai Chi has a long history. Photos from Master Lam's collection show different masters from famous traditions, arranged around a classical Tai Chi text describing fundamental movements.*

十三勢一名長拳一名十三勢。

長拳者如長江大海滔滔不絕也十三勢
者掤攦擠按採挒肘靠進退顧盼定也掤
攦擠按即坎離震兌四正方也採挒肘靠
即乾坤艮巽四斜角也此八卦也進步退
步左顧右盼中定即金木水火土也此五
行也合而言之曰十三勢

禹襄武氏識

For further study

If you wish to advance further in the study of Chi Kung, you should try to find a qualified instructor. The following videos give instruction and demonstrations of various aspects of the Chi Kung practices taught by Master Lam.

To order these videos or to arrange an individual consultation with Master Lam, please contact him at:

The Lam Association
1 Hercules Road
London SE1 7DP
Tel/Fax: +44 (0)20 7261 9049
Mobile: +44 (0)7831 802598

For general information visit Master Lam's website at:
www.lamassociation.org

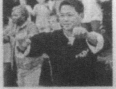

Golden Ball Tai Chi

Master Lam has distilled the essence of the arts of Tai Chi and Chi Kung into the series of exercises taught in *Tai Chi for Staying Young*. You can watch almost all these exercises on this 40-minute video. Under the direction of Master Lam, this video takes you through two 15-minute sessions of exercise that includes all the Golden Ball movements and Eight Fine Treasures presented in the book. Specifically designed for senior citizens, and filmed in London at an open-air programme taught by Master Lam, this video is the essential companion to *Tai Chi for Staying Young*.

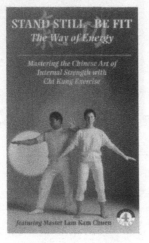

Stand Still – Be Fit

This is a series of ten-minute television programmes, each instructing you in the basic standing Chi Kung positions. Filmed on location in China and presented by Master Lam.

The Way of Power

This video is a unique presentation of the advanced practice of Da Cheng Chuan (The Great Accomplishment) for which the standing Chi Kung positions are the foundation. Filmed on location in China and London, it features both Master Lam and Professor Yu Yong-Nian, the world's leading authority on this system.

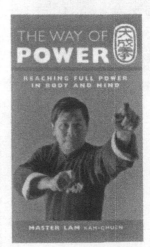

Author's acknowledgements

I have stated many times before, and would like to emphasise again, my gratitude and indebtedness to my masters and teachers for my understanding of the internal martial and healing arts. Likewise, I am truly indebted to the founders of these arts, and all the past masters who have contributed their understanding to the tradition, many of their names now lost in the passage of time. I am thankful for the depth and richness of the knowledge and practice which I have inherited.

Secondly, I would like to thank my family – especially my wife, Kai-Sin – for their support, not only for during the time of writing this book, but, for the long years of encouragement which have brought me to where I am today. I am also thankful to my three sons – Tin-Yun, Tin-Yu and Tin-Hun – who, though raised in a complex two-culture environment, have followed in the tradition of their father. They have often helped me to bridge the gap between Chinese and Western thought.

I would like to thank my students, most of whom are Westerners, for their patience and tolerance of my unusual way of teaching and my occasionally unorthodox manners. I am thankful for the openness of their minds, and those of the readers of my books in accepting these Chinese arts and philosophy.

I must also thank my students, Richard Reoch and Jane Ward, and the designer, Bridget Morley, for their assistance in producing this book. Their efforts, against the barriers of language and culture, are to be complimented. Last but not least, I would like to express my gratitude to the Managing Director, Joss Pearson, and all the staff of Gaia Books for bringing this book into print.

Finally, I am very pleased to know that there is sufficient interest amongst the public in these arts to make the publication of this book possible. I hope that this interest will be maintained, and I will, if future opportunities allow, offer more of my insights and understanding to the general public.

Master LAM Kam-Chuen

Publisher's Acknowledgements

Gaia Books would like to thank Master Lam for sharing with us his profound knowledge and experience of the Chinese internal arts, and for his tremendous energy and enthusiam. Special thanks also to Jane Ward for helping develop, with Master Lam, the programme of exercises specifically designed for senior citizens which is featured in this book.

photographic acknowledgements
Studio photography by Paul Forrester.
Location photographs: 9 Sam Scott-Hunter, 13 Lam Tin-Hun 14 Bridget Morley, 17 Lam Tin-Hun , 21 Richard Reoch.